Lessons in Leadership for
Person-Centered Elder Care

Lessons in Leadership for Person-Centered Elder Care

by

Nancy Fox

Foreword by
William H. Thomas, M.D.

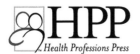

Baltimore • London • Sydney

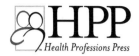

Health Professions Press, Inc.
Post Office Box 10624
Baltimore, Maryland 21285-0624

www.healthpropress.com

Interior and cover designs by Erin Geoghegan.
Manufactured in the United States of America by Integrated Books International, Dulles, VA.

Library of Congress Cataloging-in-Publication Data

Names: Fox, Nancy (Culture change consultant), author.
Title: Lessons in leadership for person-centered elder care / by Nancy Fox.
Description: Baltimore : Health Professions Press, Inc., [2017] | Includes
  bibliographical references and index.
Identifiers: LCCN 2017008812 (print) | LCCN 2017010157 (ebook) | ISBN
  9781938870729 (epub) | ISBN 9781938870606 (pbk.).
Subjects: | MESH: Health Services for the Aged | Leadership | Long-Term Care
  | Patient-Centered Care | Personal Narratives
Classification: LCC RA564.8 (ebook) | LCC RA564.8 (print) | NLM WT 31 | DDC
  362.1084/6--dc23
LC record available at https://lccn.loc.gov/2017008812

British Library Cataloguing-in-Publication data are available from the British Library.

For
the elders and their care partners

Contents

About the Author

Nancy Fox is a nationally recognized culture change consultant. She currently serves as Chief Innovation Officer for Vivage Senior Living in Lakewood, Colorado, overseeing a person-directed philosophy of care. Her career in long-term care began in the 1980s, serving at both the facility and regional levels and joining many courageous and passionate people on a journey to seek a better world for our elders and those who care for them.

Fox serves on the Leadership Team at Vivage, encouraging and informing future planning in innovative models of care, programs, and services. In 2014, she led a project in partnership with the Loveland Housing Authority to develop the first Green Houses® in Colorado. Prior to her current position, Fox served as the first Executive Director of The Eden Alternative, an international not-for-profit person-centered care organization.

In 2014, the Governor of Colorado appointed Fox to serve on the Colorado Nursing Home Innovations Grant Board. She is also a past Board Member of the Colorado Culture Change Coalition. In 2015, the Colorado Health Care Association awarded Fox the Vesta Bowden Award, its highest honor in long-term care.

A national and international speaker and educator, Fox regularly conducts training on The Eden Alternative, culture change, and leadership, and has presented at several major conferences. She is also the author of *The Journey of a Lifetime: Leadership Pathways to Culture Change in Long-Term Care* (2007). Her most important role, however, is grandmother to Nicolas and Riley.

Acknowledgments

It is unfathomable to me how to acknowledge the immeasurable number of people who have contributed in some way to this book. I have been influenced by so many people who have helped me grow as a leader and a human. This book is a confluence of many relationships, experiences, reflections, teachings, and explorations that I have had throughout my 67 years on this planet. I know that I will forget to mention many who have influenced this work, and that thought is disturbing to me. So, let me say to all of you, I am grateful for you coming into my life and helping me to grow. You have each left a handprint upon my heart.

To my children and grandchildren, who may never read this book—thanks for letting me lean on you. The mistakes I have made in "raising you" have taught me to be a better leader. My work has often taken me away from the responsibilities of being a parent and grandparent, and, consequently, I have missed many of the joys. Your acceptance of my absence has lessened that burden.

To my mentors—my father, Conde Anderson, Bill Thomas, and Jeff Jerebker—you have made my life infinitely better. I stand on your shoulders and can see farther because of you.

To the Elders—you have had to endure so much in a world that has forsaken you. I need your grace to remind me to find my own.

To those who work in a care community and give so much of themselves every day—you inspire me with your ability to love unconditionally and your courage to face the challenges of your work.

To my tribe—you have dared to seek a better way while enduring the slings and arrows of the status quo. I am honored to be among you.

To those who choose to lead—thank you for your selfless service and your willingness to learn.

To my friends and family—thank you for letting me be who I am and loving me anyway.

To Health Professions Press—thank you for publishing this work. I hope it lives up to your standards.

Then there is one who may never understand the depth of my love and gratitude. I can tell you that without her, this book would not have been written. Without her, I might not have a reason to breathe. She is the wind beneath my wings. Thank you, Sandy, for this lifetime and many others.

Foreword

One cold March morning in 1992, I sat at my kitchen table with the co-founder of The Eden Alternative, Jude Meyers Thomas. I had a pencil in hand and a yellow legal pad in front of me. Jude and I had written down nine principles that we thought should guide the nascent Eden Alternative movement. We both felt that something important was missing. As we reflected on the "missing principle," we looked back on our successes and disappointments. It soon became clear to us that success in creating a vibrant person-centered culture depended mightily on leadership. We had Eden's tenth principle: "Wise leadership is the lifeblood of any struggle against the three plagues (loneliness, helplessness, and boredom). For it, there can be no substitute." Our experience over the decades of work since that morning has confirmed and re-confirmed the truth of that assertion. Leadership is, and will always remain, essential to the work of fostering person-centered cultures.

The first book in the field of long-term care that successfully explored the cultural terrain that lies beyond policies and procedures was Bruce Vladek's *Unloving Care: The Nursing Home Tragedy* (1980). In Vladek's view, long-term care was destined to struggle against endemic shortcomings related to quality and resident and family satisfaction, because "good facilities do not drive poor ones out of business, nor is there a direct correlation between quality and price." Without the discipline of a functioning marketplace that features a range of competing service options, long-term care's industry standards became almost exclusively concerned with inputs (staffing, physical facilities) and process (paperwork).

At the most practical level, outcomes came to matter little, or not at all.

The person-centered care movement, which burst forth in the 1990s, sought to address these shortcomings by articulating (and promoting) powerful intrinsic motivations that could function in place of the missing extrinsic markers that could define success at the personal level. Nancy Fox was a prominent early leader of this movement and served for many years as the Executive Director of The Eden Alternative. She guided the organization's expansion from a small nonprofit into a thriving global nonprofit. She has taught, mentored, and inspired long-term care leaders all over the world for more than two decades. From the beginning she has understood and wielded stories and storytelling as powerful culture (and career) making tools. It is experience that has taught her that while systems can enforce compliance with standards, full participation in a vibrant person-centered culture requires a purely individual commitment. The former can be demanded, the latter must be earned.

Happily, this book uses a series of compelling stories to illuminate highly practical lessons in person-centered leadership. The stories serve to illuminate the myths, and the truths, of daily practice in long-term care and offer the reader practical strategies for building a culture that is solidly founded on the principles of well-being, while also delivering superior clinical and financial outcomes.

Lessons in Leadership for Person-Centered Elder Care should be seen as a particularly effective bookend to Vladek's (now out of print) classic. In my view, the field has long needed, and now has, a practical and superbly well-informed (and proudly personal) perspective on person-centered leadership that can help us shape the next 40 years of long-term care.

William H. Thomas, M.D.
Co-founder, The Eden Alternative®

Preface

Person-Centered Leadership
Elevating the Art

I must be willing to give up what I am in order to become what I will be.

—Albert Einstein

In 2007, I wrote a book about the leadership pathways a formal leader in long-term care must take to make the leap from an institutional model to a person-centered model of care. The title of the book, *The Journey of a Lifetime: Leadership Pathways to Culture Change in Long-Term Care,* expresses my belief that leadership is a lifelong journey of self-reflection and self-growth. It also reflected my conviction that there are certain beliefs and behaviors, or "paths," that a leader must take to lead an organization through cultural transformation.

I believe the concepts in that book are still valid for, and important to, a journey of transformation. I found myself compelled to write again about the same topic, not only because my journey of growth has continued, but also because it seems everywhere I look, I find formal leaders who continue to try to lead from old, institutional habits and expect a different outcome. The institutional creep is so strong, I even find myself being sucked back into its clutches time and time again. Dr. William H. Thomas, one of my mentors, calls the institution "a dragon sleeping in the corner." He reminds us that if we feed the dragon, it will wake up. The most powerful forms of dragon food, I believe, are the attitudes, beliefs, assumptions, and behaviors of formal leaders. Until we change ourselves, until we find new thinking that leads to new behaviors, we are destined as a profession to remain stuck in the past, doomed by our own inability to change.

Do not get me wrong: there have been enormous changes in long-term care since I wrote my first book. New physical designs, organizational architecture, tools, programs, and systems have all led to improvements in quality of care and quality of life for our residents. Yet, we as leaders in long-term care are still in crisis, and we continue to grapple with many of the same problems we have had for years. More important, the overall perception of nursing homes remains negative. We are now facing an all-out assault from state and federal governmental agencies. There is an ill-informed belief that we do not need skilled nursing homes, except for short-term rehabilitation services, and that most residents of long-term care would be better served (at a lower cost, supposedly) in their own homes. I believe the choice for long-term care providers is clear. We can continue to try to "improve" the quality of our services and risk the fate of the best buggy whip makers of the previous century, or we can embrace the evolution of our work and ourselves as leaders to position ourselves for a future that desperately needs us, not in our current identity, but as an evolved entity. Evolution builds on pre-existing capabilities. So all of the gains and improvements we have made in long-term care since the 1980s are not lost. In fact, those very gains have positioned us for the evolution that we must undertake to survive into the future. If we do not evolve, then we will surely face extinction.

The kind of transformation required begins with us, the formal leaders in long-term care. We need to ask ourselves the same question that Albert Einstein asked of himself: "Am I willing to give up what I am in order to become what I will be?" If you are reading this book, then you have at least considered that choice.

So, here is my current thinking and the premise for this book. Leadership is an art, not a science. As with any art, there is an understanding that it requires practice, study, growth, learning, and diligence, all in an effort to approach mastery—and all the while knowing that complete mastery is unachievable. As with any art, no matter how long or hard we study, there will always be room for more growth and learning. But there is also a science that we must understand in order to elevate that art.

Think of any art. What is the science the artist must use to approach mastery in that art? Painters, no matter the medium, must understand the science of mathematics as well as perspective, composition, color, value and hue, and light and dark. Photography is an art whose science has changed dramatically over the years, most recently with digital photography. Now, instead of a dark room, photographers use a computer to enhance their art. But despite the technological advances, much of the science of photography remains the same, such as light and shadow, composition, and depth of field. For the art of music, as with painting, regardless of the instrument you play or if your voice is your instrument, there is much science. Here we find mathematics again with beat and rhythm and scales spanning an octave. There is the science of sound with melody and pitch, harmony, and timbre. And no matter which instrument you play or what style of music you produce, the science is important. If you do not believe me, try listening to someone singing off key.

I once toured a Van Gogh exhibit where I learned how he would weave together different strands of colored yarn to determine which colors were complementary to each other. I read how he studied complementary colors and applied them next to each other instead of blending them together to get the effect he wanted. He had learned that when you blend colors together, they can become muddy and lose their vibrancy. From the exhibit, I was able to trace the path of Van Gogh's growth toward mastery through his paintings over time and through his study and use of science to elevate his art.

Every artist uses science as a means of elevating his or her art. If the artist does not first understand the science, the path to mastery is illusive. If that is true, then what is the science that we must use to elevate the art of leadership?

As leaders in long-term care, we must use the sciences of human behavior, the brain, social systems, and organizational behavior. Even the science of quantum physics can help us.

Leaders in many other industries have successfully been using these sciences for decades. Yet, many long-term care leaders continue to cling to outdated management and human resource practices that make working in care communities almost insufferable. This is not because we are bad people, but because we are stuck in a punitive paradigm where risk and innovation are choked out by fear and threats. We are allowing our old perceptions, our old beliefs, and our own fears to blind us to a new way, a way that is solidly based in research over the past 40 to 50 years. This research is now leading us to new ways of thinking and new ways of behaving as leaders. But it will only lead us if we are willing to let go of our own fears, let go of who we were so that we can become who we must be to lead long-term care into the future.

Throughout the book, I share some of the science I have learned in pursuit of the art of leadership. I do not claim to be a psychologist, neurologist, sociologist, or organizational specialist, or to even approach a deep understanding of these sciences. I am just a long-term care leader who has had the incredible fortune of being a part of a social movement to change our industry. What I can share is not only how I and other long-term care leaders have drawn upon the lessons we have learned (mostly through our mistakes and the eventual shifts we have had to make in ourselves to lead an organization through the change process), but also what we have learned from other leaders and through the dedicated pursuit of knowledge. I translate these lessons into actual shifts in thinking and behavior that are needed for a person-centered leader embarking on the journey away from the institutional model. These shifts are essential in creating a sustainable transformation and culture of growth in which each person contributes to a caring community.

I SIT AT THE FEET OF MY MASTERS

In many traditions, it is said that a moment spent at the feet of a Master is worth a lifetime of learning from books or school. I understand and appreciate this belief, for I have been blessed to sit at the feet of many Masters throughout my life. In my acknowledgments for this book, I name a few of them. But I mention this here because I believe that all of us who have been called to lead care communities have been duly blessed. Each and every day, through our sacred work, we come in contact with Masters. For each of us, these Masters may come in different forms. They may come in the form of a superior who guides and mentors us, a family member who complains to us, a hands-on caregiver who amazes us with her capacity to give, or our favorite elder who shares a laugh with us each day. I do know we all share some of the same Masters. They come in the form of those who challenge us the most, who cause us the most angst, who do not fit into the mold we want them to fit into, who we struggle to help and understand, who we lose sleep over, and who make us look deep inside ourselves, searching for the answer, questioning ourselves, challenging our own beliefs and attitudes, seeking a better way. These people are our greatest teachers, our greatest Masters. And in long-term care, we are blessed with many of these Masters. Some days they seem to be everywhere. Are we listening and learning from them?

Through the process of writing this book, I know that I will continue to grow myself toward the mastery of leadership. If that growth can help me better learn the lessons of my Masters, then I will have been successful. If you are reading this book, our journeys will become entwined. Through that process, if you can gain even a small kernel of insight or growth that aids you in the important and noble work you do, then I will be thankful.

A WORD ABOUT LANGUAGE

In this book, I have chosen to use the term *person-centered* to describe a cultural transformation away from the institutional framework and way of being in long-term care toward a truly caring community. The culture change movement has struggled to choose one term in describing the new way. Some use *person-centered*, while others think *person-directed* is more appropriate. I have even heard arguments for using *person-directed living* instead of *person-directed care,* as well as *self-directed care* and *self-directed living.* I do not think anyone has suggested we call the new way "self-centered care," but that might be an interesting model.

I understand the importance of language in creating a world. The institutional model gave us some horrendous language that people outside of long-term care would not understand. Have you ever been at a party and had someone leave the table to "toilet" themselves? Have you ever heard someone refer to their grandmother as "the feeder?" We need to change our language to change our behavior.

I have chosen *person-centered* to refer to a new way of thinking and behaving that will lead to the transformation of our long-term care communities into places where people want to live and work. Places where everyone can experience well-being. That is it. Plain and simple.

I am living for the day when the new way becomes *the* way and we do not need a term to define it. Achieving that vision will require a lot more people acting as leaders. Thank you for being one of them.

CHAPTER 1

How It Is

Three Stories & One Myth

LESSON 1
Sanibel Island

The sea does not reward those who are too anxious, too greedy, or too impatient. To dig for treasures shows not only impatience and greed, but lack of faith. Patience, patience, patience, is what the sea teaches. Patience and faith. One should lie empty, open, choiceless as a beach— waiting for a gift from the sea.

—Anne Morrow Lindbergh, author and aviator

SUMMER, 2003

I was tired. No, not just tired, but weary; the kind of bone-weary that those who travel for a living understand better than most. The work was good. No, not just good, but fulfilling. So my spirit was full, at the same time my body was fatigued and needed a rest. In 2001, I had begun my work as the first executive director of The Eden Alternative®. My personal journey of transformation, however, had begun 5 years earlier in 1996, when I was the administrator of a skilled nursing facility in central Texas. I was fortunate in the spring of that year to have attended the very first Eden Alternative® training ever held, and immediately put those valuable lessons to work. For the next 5 years, my organization underwent a transformation from a traditional (institutional) model of care to an Eden Alternative, or person-centered, model of care. That experience was enlightening and inspiring, but also exhausting. If anyone ever tells you that cultural transformation of a care community is easy, run as fast as you can. They are not telling you the truth. As Anne Morrow Lindbergh expresses, the treasures of culture change, like those from the sea, require patience and faith. And like the treasures of the sea, they are a rare and wondrous gift.

I knew deep in my soul that these were gifts that must be shared with the world. So when the opportunity arrived to bring the message of The Eden Alternative to the world, I happily accepted that challenge. But now I needed a respite. For me, the most restful and renewing place is the beach. I grew up going to the beach, and some of my fondest memories as a child are memories of sand and surf and seashells. I love nature and the gifts that the sea offers up each night to those who are patient and have faith.

One of the best shelling beaches in the United States can be found just off the southwestern coast of Florida on a tiny island in the Gulf of Mexico. Sanibel Island is a small, quiet community of less than 7,000 people, but it attracts thousands of tourists each year who come to comb the beaches in search of beautiful treasures from the sea. It is one of my favorite places.

On this trip, I could not wait to get to the beach and let the stress slowly leave my body. On our first morning there, we walked to a local diner for breakfast. We wanted to avoid the tourists, so we asked the locals for the best and quickest way to a quiet beach. We were directed down a small caliche lane. As we entered the lane, we could see a patch of blue beckoning us about a quarter mile away. I was already beginning to relax with the smell of salt in the air and the sun on my back.

About halfway down the lane, I noticed an elder man standing by the edge of the road in front of a house. My elder-radar immediately went into effect, as I began surveying the scene ahead of me. This thin, frail gentleman must have been in his nineties. He was leaning shakily on a cane, and with his other hand at only waist height, he appeared to be calling us to him with his hand motions. He was unshaven and dressed in loose clothing. I approached him, smiling. He said something to me, but I could not make out what it was. Instinctively, I knew something was not right with this scene. So I came closer. I had to put my ear next to his face to hear what he was saying.

"She fell and can't get up."

I knew immediately one of two things was happening here: there was someone hurt in the house, or this man was confused and should not be out by the street alone. Either scenario required our further investigation.

I asked, "Do you need some help?" He nodded. I then asked, "Do you need me to come inside with you?" He nodded again. So I took his arm, and we began a treacherous journey across an entire front yard full of small stones. How he traversed the yard to get to the road, I will never know. On our way, he said, "No one would stop." I reassured him that we were here now and would help.

As my foot hit the front steps of the house, I could hear her moans. We found her lying on the linoleum floor in front of the kitchen sink. She was crying in pain. There had been several times in my life that I was immensely thankful that my partner is a nurse. This was yet another one. I had to step over the prone woman to get to the phone. My partner, Sandy, immediately bent down to attend to her.

I dialed 911. As the phone was ringing, I looked at the man who was standing on the other side of the woman and asked him for his address. The woman answered, "107 Buttonwood Lane." I asked the man, "What is your name?" Between moans, the woman answered, "Appleby. Abigail and Henry Appleby." I relayed the information to the operator and requested an ambulance. Sandy was comforting the woman and trying to keep her still.

When I hung up, I asked if there was a son or daughter I could call. Abigail answered, "No." I asked if there was a relative I could call. Through a cry of pain, Abigail answered again, "There's no one." I asked if there was a neighbor or friend to call. "No one," came the reply. "How about a minister or other acquaintance?" I asked. "There's no one," she said. Those three words rang coldly in my heart. But I did not have time at that moment to consider their import.

Instead, my administrator training kicked in and I began to assess the scene before me. Abigail was lying in pain on the cold floor in a threadbare cotton housecoat. Beside her lay a worn bath mat. I picked it up and found the rubber backing had worn away. Breakfast dishes were still in the sink. Abigail had become incontinent either before or after her fall; a small pool of urine was beside her, the bottom of her housecoat soaked.

I took Henry by the arm and led him to a chair in the breakfast room where he could still watch over her, but be safe from falling on the wet floor. Her cries continued. And in that moment, I realized that the cries we were hearing were certainly from the pain of her injury (most likely a broken hip), but more than that, these were cries from the pain of the human spirit. Abigail's world had just collapsed in on her. Here was a 90-something-year-old woman caring for her husband, who was living with dementia. She was trying desperately to hang onto the life they had made together. And in the blink of an eye, in less time than it takes to wash a dirty coffee cup, that life just came crashing down. *And there was no one to call.* I knew in that instant that she was crying for her loss and for the certainty of a future she did not want to imagine. And although I managed to maintain my own composure, in that moment I felt her pain, and my heart wept at what I was witnessing.

The paramedics arrived with a stretcher. Two nice young men took over ministrations of Abigail. I sat next to Henry and reassured him that he would go with her to the hospital. Then SHE burst into the room with such force, it startled me. She must have been all of 25 years old, but this EMT commanded everyone's attention just by the way she entered the room. Cocky would be an understatement. She pushed the young men out of the way, bent down, and touched Abigail's hip. Realizing that Abigail had become incontinent, the woman let loose with the most degrading "UGH!" I have ever heard. She then backed away and had the young men once again attend to Abigail. She made a call on her walkie-talkie and then she barked some orders to the young men.

I asked to speak with her, as she was obviously in charge. I told her that we were vacationing here and were just passing by when we saw Henry and came into the house to find Abigail. I informed her that we had inquired about relatives and friends, but there was no one to call. I then suggested that she take Henry with them to the hospital. She looked over at Henry sitting quietly, staring at the young men working with Abigail. And then she said very loudly, loud enough for everyone in that room and the house next door to hear, "We are not babysitters!"

Now, I am a peaceful person, but at that moment, it took every ounce of restraint I had in me not to yank her by her cute little ponytail out into the yard and smack her. Instead, I said, "There are social workers at the hospital who can get Henry to a safe place." Her response was, "They are not babysitters either." I then pulled her aside, out of earshot, and told her that I was a nursing home administrator and had assessed this situation. It was obvious that Henry was living with dementia, and she was about to take his only caregiver with her in an ambulance. She could either take him with her now and make sure he was in a safe place, or she could come back in a few hours and pick him up in an ambulance, and that would be on *her* head. She then asked me why I did not take him. I told her I wished I could, but if she had been listening the first time, she would know there is no one to call. I helped Henry to the ambulance, and off they went.

Sandy and I continued our walk to the beach, but I could not find solace there. I told Sandy that I needed to go back to our room. I understood why Abigail was in so much pain. For the first time in my life, I got it. At that moment, I laid "empty, open and choiceless as the beach," awaiting the gift.

Once we returned to our room, I took out my computer and tried to find an Eden Alternative registered home anywhere in the area. I did not have much hope, for at that time, when it came to culture change and person-centered care, Florida was a wasteland, other than a few bright spots. But I had to try. If I could find one in the area, then I could ask someone on staff at the home to go to the hospital and check on Abigail and Henry. And, maybe, I could have a moment of peace, knowing that they were in good hands. But it was to no avail. I was distraught.

Sandy and I returned to the beach, and I went through the motions of hunting for seashells. I assumed the "Sanibel stoop" as the locals call it—shoulders hunched, bent over watching the sand. But my mind was anything but peaceful. I kept asking, "How could this happen?" Sanibel Island is not some big metropolis where elders can become isolated and forgotten. This was a sleepy little seaside village. Yet for Abigail and Henry, it might as well have been the middle of New York City. Their words kept resounding in my mind:

"There is no one to call."

Then there was the absolute disdain shown by the young woman whose job it was to care for people. How does that happen? When did our elders become invisible? And should they require some kind of help, when did it become appropriate to call them babies and sneer at their discomfort and the embarrassment of incontinence? Of all the beaches in the world, why did I walk down that lane on that day? My mind was reeling.

And then it hit me.

I had come to Sanibel looking for a treasure, a gift from the sea. I thought it would come in the form of rest and relaxation and, if I was lucky, a beautiful and rare seashell. But that was not to be. My gift from the sea came in the form of two elders, Abigail and Henry. Their gift was much more precious than the ones I had imagined. They gave me the gift of looking through their eyes at a world that has forsaken its elders, and in doing so, has lost one of its most priceless treasures.

Had this happened in New York City, or Houston, or Los Angeles, or any other large city, I might have missed the point. But, it happened in a sleepy seaside village, the last place on earth you would think elders could disappear. There was no one to call. And if it could happen here, it could happen anywhere. Abigail and Henry showed me how an ageist culture was failing all of us. It certainly failed them. But it had also failed that young, insolent EMT. She, too, was suffering because we have lost our elders. I knew then that what we were fighting went far beyond the walls of the nursing home. It went to the farthest reaches of our nation, our world. The loss of our elders was hurting us all.

But this is not the only gift Abigail and Henry gave me that day. Through her cries of pain, Abigail showed me what I should have seen long ago. She showed me why people do not like nursing homes. I am a nursing home administrator. I know the kind of caring people that work in nursing homes. I know how hard they work and how much they adore their elders. Why, then, do more than 30% of seriously ill people say they would rather die than live in a nursing home (Gilbert, 1997)?

If you go to a provider association meeting or conference, you can discover all of the advancements in quality that have been made over the last 30–40 years. The mantra is quality—quality initiatives, quality measures, quality improvement, quality care. Nursing homes are highly regulated by governmental agencies in an effort to ensure safety, quality, and residents' rights. If that is true, then why do our elders still say, "Whatever you do, don't put me in a nursing home"?

In their decades-long quest for quality, nursing home providers and owners have failed to ask themselves an important question. Abigail and Henry showed me the right question. As Abigail lay on that cold, hard floor writhing in pain, I finally understood the question: *What are they afraid of?*

In that moment, I felt Abigail's fear, and I knew the answer. And I cringed. It is why I needed to try to find an Eden Alternative home for her and Henry. I knew what was in store for them. I knew her fear in the deepest part of my soul. She was not afraid that she and Henry would not receive the best medical care available.

That worry probably never crossed her mind. She was not afraid that Henry would not get his medications on time or three nutritionally sound meals and a snack per physician's orders. She was not even worried that there would not be a van to take her to the grocery store. Abigail's fear, and the fear of every other elder living in an ageist world, was the loss of her identity, security, autonomy, meaning, connectedness, growth, and joy. That fear was so great that it kept her and Henry isolated from their community, struggling to maintain their dignity and clinging to each other in a desperate battle against all odds—the odds of time.

I will never know what became of Abigail and Henry. But to this day, they and elders like them are why I work hard trying to share their wisdom with others. It is why I work to bring a message of hope rather than despair to our elders. For I know that what Abigail feared was a symptom of the institutional model of care. And I know that when we understand the power of community in a human life and work hard to transform our institutions into truly caring communities, then our elders will not need to fear anymore.

LESSON 2
Parkview Care Center

Only he who attempts the absurd is capable of achieving the impossible.

—Miguel de Unamuno, writer and philosopher

SUMMER, 2008

The irony of the name, Parkview Care Center, struck me the moment I arrived on Arkansas Street in Denver. There is nothing even vaguely resembling a park anywhere near Arkansas Street. There is cracked asphalt and concrete, grass and weeds strangling through the crevices. There are dilapidated apartment buildings, old retail stores, falling down fences, and dirty streets, but no park. And not even any place to park.

I was warned before my first visit to Parkview. Make sure you do not leave anything visible in your vehicle, or it will be gone when you come out. "Welcome to Denver," I thought. I had just taken a new position with Piñon Management, and Parkview Care Center was one of the care communities I would oversee.

As I walked toward the front door that first day, I had a hard time believing that this community had been under the management of Piñon for the past 2 years. Not because it was an old building, built in the 1960s. Piñon managed plenty of those. Not because it was in the "hood." Piñon managed another community half a block down Arkansas Street. Not because it cared for the chronically mentally ill. Piñon had several other communities that did a remarkable job caring for what I call "the throw away people"—those for whom no one else wants to provide care. The reason I struggled was because I had been in other Piñon communities similar to this one and had found life, love, and leadership.

I have visited and worked with dozens of care communities in my career. So many that it only takes me a few minutes, sometimes less than a minute, to assess the "feel" or climate of a home.

I understand the impact that leadership has on organizational climate and culture. And I know how climate and culture impact the lives of the people who live and work in those care communities. I knew right away that what I was feeling before I even approached the front door of Parkview was caused by a lack of leadership in that community.

I stopped on my walk in to pick up the trash and cigarette butts I found in the flower beds and on the sidewalk. The front entrance looked like it had not been touched in 50 years: faded, cracked paint; no flowers; dead, overgrown plants; and trash, just what you might expect in that neighborhood if you did not know this was a Piñon home (Hint #1). As I entered the building, there were residents sitting in wheelchairs lined up along the walls. Some of them had assumed the institutional model "slump." (Not to be confused with the "Sanibel stoop.") No one greeted me (Hint #2). The interior décor (walls, paint, lighting, furnishings) was out of the 1960s (Hint #3). I asked where I might find the administrator and was told, "In her office" (Hint #4). No one offered to show me where her office was, so I ventured out on my own (Hint #5). No one I passed was smiling (Hint #6). The door to the office was closed (Hint #7). Inside the "office" (a former resident room), I found both the administrator and director of nursing, their desks and every available surface piled with papers (Hint #8).

So I had left my car less than 2 minutes ago, and I already know, without having seen one single outcome, that this was a home in trouble. And I already know that the problem lies in the office I was standing in. The problem was not the types of residents, the age of the building or décor, the location of the community, or the staff. The problem is where it always lies with the leadership (or lack thereof) in a care community.

As I came to discover later, this home was indeed in serious trouble. But that had never stopped Piñon before. This company was known for taking over the management of some of the most challenging and troubled communities and successfully turning them around by introducing a person-centered model of care and leadership. In more than 2 years, however, this home had not paid one dime in management fees to Piñon, and currently owed more than $700,000 just to Piñon alone. This did not take into account the other accounts payable. The money Piñon planned on using to upgrade the interior of the home quickly vanished in addressing more pressing needs, such as furnaces and roofs that had not been touched in 50 years. The current stove was on its last leg, as well as every other piece of equipment in the building. While just down the street, less than a block away, was a sister community that was thriving under the direction of a person-centered leader.

I believe in growing people, so we gave it a try at Parkview. Not just that day, but for the next 2 months. Every suggestion I made, every question I asked, was met with the same excuse: "We can't because . . . " (Hint #9). And every time I visited the home, I found the same issues (Hint #10).

Ample research comparing high-performing nursing homes with low-performing homes has repeatedly shown the impact that leadership, especially at the level of administrator and director of nursing, has on quality in all areas, from financial to clinical to human resource management.

In one of these studies conducted through the University of Nebraska, researchers compared extreme case examples of both high- and low-performing nursing homes (Forbes-Thompson, Leiker, & Bleich, 2007). Data were collected through more than 100 hours of observation, 70 formal interviews, numerous informal interviews, and document review. Findings showed that formal leaders in the high-performing homes "behaved consistently with the nursing home's stated and lived mission by fostering connectivity among staff" (relationships); maintained "ample information flow" (communication); and incorporated the "use of cognitive diversity" (inviting differing opinions based on how we think differently). In contrast, leadership in low-performing homes behaved disharmoniously with the stated mission, which ultimately "confused and eroded trust and relationships among staff members, contributed to poor communication, and fostered role isolation and discontinuity in resident care."

The study suggested that

> an overuse of mechanistic, linear command-and-control approaches to improving care, such as punitive measures to insist on regulatory compliance, will do little to ultimately improve care. Rather, relationship-centered leadership that embraces co-management and mutual shaping of resident care complements doing the right thing for residents from

a values-based shared experience. Examples of practice implications included developing a strong, coherent organizational mission; having fewer, more flexible rules to foster creativity; and allowing lateral decision making. (Forbes-Thompson, Leiker, & Bleich, 2007, p. 341)

So, my suggestion for improving Parkview was easily formed. Find a new administrator. The current administrator is either incapable of or unwilling to grow, which is not only contributing to, but also causing this community's low performance. It is rare that an effective formal leader has to terminate anyone. If we are truly acting as leaders, the person we are leading will already know upon termination that she has not been successful in her role. In this case, the administrator resigned, and we replaced her with a proven person-centered leader.

This home was the most unlikely place for a person-centered model of care to take hold. Half of the residents lived with chronic mental illness. Many of them had never before had a home, literally. They had lived on the streets. Many exhibited expressions of unmet needs (behaviors) that required ample staff attention. Half of them were old and frail. The vast majority were Hispanic and spoke only Spanish. Many of them lived with comorbidities and complications from lifelong unhealthy lifestyles. Ninety-five percent of the residents were Medicaid recipients.

One of Piñon's long-tenured administrators had been promoted to a position at the corporate offices. She volunteered to return as an administrator to turn Parkview around. One of our corporate social workers who wanted to train as an administrator joined her as assistant administrator and resident services director. The first step the new administrator took was to implement two daily community meetings, one in English and one in Spanish. She wanted to bring the voice of the residents into the daily life of the community. She was sending a very loud message that their voices counted. The second step was to take her morning clinical meetings to the neighborhoods. (A key principle in providing person-centered care is to create real home. In that vein, Piñon, as well as other communities that embrace culture change, use the term *neighborhood* as opposed to *hall* or *unit*.) This home already had consistent assignment of staff on two separate neighborhoods. (It had been a Piñon home for 2 years, so some of the best practices of person-centered care were already in place.) Through this new practice of engaging the hands-on staff in communication and process improvement, the new administrator was sending a very loud message that the staff's voice counted. She was systematically dismantling the current ruling structure and beginning to place more decision-making authority in the hands of the residents and those closest to them.

She began growing a cohesive leadership team in part by initiating learning circles and huddles (see Lesson # 30). She deployed all of the resources that the corporation offered her, through both best practices and consultants. But it was not easy. The climate of the home was still very cold from years of institutional leadership practices. Pessimism, cynicism, and stinginess abounded at Parkview. Regardless, this seasoned, person-centered leader continued to grow herself as well as her staff. And over time she learned some hard lessons in this community. One of the hardest was how she needed to make herself vulnerable in order to gain trust.

In the end, all of her efforts paid off. Figures 2.1, 2.2, and 2.3 show just a few of the empirical results she attained. The financial and regulatory improvements were accompanied by improvements in clinical indicators, staff retention, and customer satisfaction. But equally important were the stories of residents who found a true home and community. As one of Parkview's residents commented, "This is the first home I have ever had."

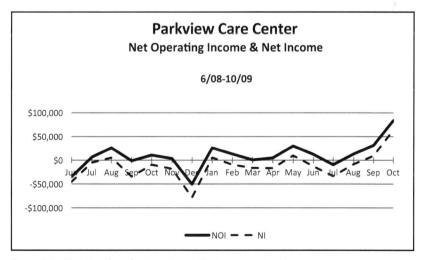

Figure 2.1. Parkview Care Center net operating income and net income.

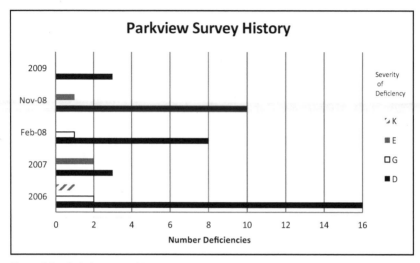

Figure 2.2. Parkview survey history.

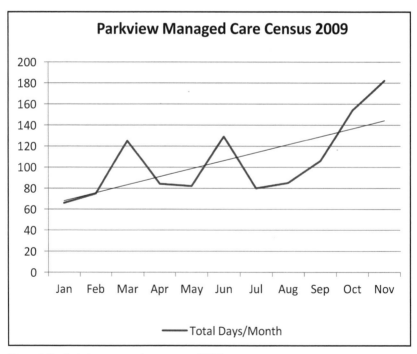

Figure 2.3. Parkview managed care census (2009).

These successes, however, were not easily earned. They required leaders who were willing to hold themselves accountable. I happened to be in one learning circle at Parkview with managers and staff when a neighborhood nurse commented that management, including the administrator and the owner of Piñon, were stingy and did not care. I personally stopped being shocked by these kinds of perceptions years ago, but as I looked over at the administrator, I could see both astonishment and bewilderment on her face.

I started sending her a telepathic message: "Do not take this personally! Do not get defensive!" It is very difficult as a leader, when you are working as hard as you can to make a better world for everyone, to hear others' perceptions of you that are not consistent with the way you see yourself. But I understood the power of context and past experiences in shaping one's perceptions. I only hoped that this administrator would also recognize this. So I quickly asked the nurse, "Can you please share with us a reason why you believe that?"

She told us that there was a suction machine in the dining room that had not been functioning properly for 2 months. She was outraged that we would allow that to continue, putting the residents at risk. I looked at the administrator. Her jaw had dropped to her chest. She was unaware of this. I looked at the director of nursing—same expression. Come to find out, the suction machine was a rented piece of equipment. All it took was one, simple phone call to replace it.

It was clear to me that the administration, corporation, and ownership of this home were caring and generous. Yet, a breakdown in communication, false perceptions, and assumptions on the part of everyone involved had led to a potentially dangerous situation.

The sad reality is that this story (or some version of this story) could be told of 16,000 nursing homes across the country. All the more reason why we need a new kind of leadership, one that is person-centered and based on the science of what we know about human behavior, the inner working of our brains, how we behave based on context, what motivates us as human beings, and how we relate to each other. We need the science to elevate the art.

In response to this event, I wrote a story that we use at Vivage Senior Living in our Neighborhood Guide curriculum for developing self-managed teams to illustrate how assumptions hurt us and put elders at risk. It teaches both managers and hands-on staff how to hold themselves accountable by breaking down the walls between each constituency to ensure the well-being of the elders. It is called "The Farmer and the Hoe-maker," and it is included at the end of this lesson as a tool for you to use.

Parkview Care Center is a testament to the power of formal leaders in making a better world against all odds. As Cervantes reminds us, "In order to attain the impossible, one must attempt the absurd." And this is what the leaders at Parkview did. They attempted the absurd by creating a caring community in the unlikeliest of settings, in an underfunded system, with some of the most interesting and diverse characters as residents, blending young and old as well as those who only spoke either English or Spanish. The community has only continued to grow and improve, even after the administrator left and the assistant administrator took over. So the cultural transformation has been sustainable. It was not charismatic leadership that changed this home. It was person-centered leadership. And person-centered leadership is something we can all learn.

I only wish Abigail and Henry could have benefitted from this kind of caring community.

The Farmer and the Hoe-maker

Once upon a time, a long, long time ago, in a small village on the western slope of the Rocky Mountains, there lived a poor farmer and his family. Year after year, the farmer worked every day from sunrise to sunset on his small patch of land, trying to eke out enough food to sustain his family through the cold winters until he could plant again. The only tool the poor farmer had to aid him in his daily labor was a rusty and worn hoe he had inherited from his grandfather. Year after year, the poor farmer used the old hoe to remove all the rocks from the soil so he could plant his meager garden. Each year the hoe became even rustier and more worn.

Coincidentally, in this same small village lived the best hoe-maker in the world. The man was renowned far and wide for his ability to make the most beautiful and most productive hoes ever made. Just when you thought there was no way to improve on his creations, the hoe-maker would make an even better hoe. Farmers would come from miles around each year to buy one of his hoes. These hoes were not only beautiful, but the farmers said that they could do twice as much work in half the time using one of these hoes.

This hoe-maker had great hoe-making skills, that is true, but he also possessed a most generous heart. Each year, at the end of the growing season, at the annual harvest festival, he would give away his remaining stock of hoes to the poor farmers who could not afford to purchase them. Then, through the long, cold winters, he would make a new stock of his latest creations.

The hoe-maker and his family lived on a small farm outside of town. Every day on his way into his shop, he would pass by the poor farmer's land and see the farmer working hard removing the many rocks that would surface in the soil. Every day he would wave to the poor farmer and tip his hat in greeting. And every day the farmer would look up from his labors and wave to the hoe-maker. Then each afternoon, on his way home for supper, the hoe-maker would again pass by the poor farmer's land and see him still working away. And each evening the two exchanged greetings again as the sun slowly set in the west.

On some of these occasions, the hoe-maker would wonder silently why the poor farmer continued to use his old, rusty hoe when all he needed to do was ask and the hoe-maker would gladly give him a wonderful new hoe that would make his labors easier. "He must be a stubborn young man," the hoe-maker thought. And on some of these

(continued)

(continued)

occasions, the poor farmer would wonder why the hoe-maker did not offer to give him a new hoe. Couldn't he see how he struggled day after day with the old one? "He must be a greedy old man," the poor farmer thought.

Day after day, year after year, their paths crossed twice each day. And day after day, year after year, the poor farmer struggled. Until one day, his rusty old hoe broke, and all he was left with was the rusty blade. So the poor farmer had to get on his hands and knees and use the blade of the broken hoe to try to till his soil. And that winter, there were some nights his family went hungry. That year, as the hoe-maker passed by the poor farmer's land, he would shake his head and think, "What a shame. His stubbornness will be his demise." And that year, when the poor farmer looked up from his work to see the hoe-maker passing by, he did not wave but only became angrier and angrier as he cursed the hoe-maker's greed that was hurting his family.

Then one day, as the poor farmer knelt on his hands and knees and brought the blade of his rusty hoe down, it struck a rock and shattered. Without any tools, the poor farmer then had to use his bare hands to try to till his soil. And that year, the farmer was unable to grow enough food for his family to last through the long, cold winter. When the spring came again, as the hoe-maker passed by the poor farmer's land, he was surprised to see no one tending the fields. And as he passed he shook his head, and said, "What a shame."

***Whenever you share a story as a learning tool, be sure to discuss the story and how it applies to our work by asking some follow-up questions. Here are a few to use with this story:

1. That was a sad story, wasn't it? Did it have to end that way?
2. Who was at fault in that story?
3. Were the farmer and the hoe-maker bad people?
4. What could either of them have done that might have changed the outcome of this story?
5. How is this story like a nursing home?
6. What can we do to make sure this kind of thing does not happen here?

LESSON 3
Her Name Was Grace

Motherhood: all love begins and ends here.

—Robert Browning, poet and playwright

WINTER, 2014

It was Christmas, and I was visiting my mother in her home town in south Texas, as I did every Christmas. Suffice it to say, my mother and I were not close. We talked on the phone about once a month and visited during holidays. This year, the nagging started before I could get into her house. She did not like my hair. On this Christmas, I am not 13 years old; I am 63. Yet, in those 63 years, I do not believe I had yet met my mother's expectations of me. Still, she was my mother. And all that I had learned throughout my life and my career implored me to honor and respect her. I could intellectualize her criticisms of me and, most of the time, not take them personally. I learned that skill from my father. But he was not around anymore to remind me. On this Christmas, the criticisms stung more than usual and were coming in waves. It seemed I was unable to do anything right, even properly putting the ketchup back where it belonged.

If you were to have ever met my mother, you would think that the previous paragraph was fantasy. She was a remarkable, beautiful, and charming woman. She was adored by everyone who knew her. On this Christmas, she was 89 years old, but to look at her, you might have guessed she was 69. She took pride in her youthful appearance. She was a caretaker. She took care of herself and her home in meticulous fashion. She surrounded herself with beauty. She took care of her children and her grandchildren and her great grandchildren. She took care of her garden. She took care of her friends and other relatives. She took care of her church. And she was loved. I loved her and knew she loved me. But for this Christmas, the criticisms were more than I could handle. I understood that her very identity was wrapped up in her ability to host a beautiful holiday meal, complete with all the china and sterling and crystal. I understood her need for every detail to be perfect. That was who she was: the perfect hostess, the ideal homemaker, the social elite.

That night, as I was lying in bed recalling the stressful day, I texted my partner, Sandy. She still has all of the texts I sent her that night and teases me about them occasionally. I am pleading with her to rescue me. I am about to commit hari-kari. If I have to stay in this house one more minute, I am going to kill myself or my mother. But that night, there was no rescuing, so I was doomed to face another day of my mother's incessant criticisms. Despite the fact that I am a highly competent professional who raised two successful and kind sons and has had a beautiful partner of almost 30 years, I am unable to complete the simplest of tasks to my mother's approval.

There is nothing like a night's sleep to bring perspective and understanding. When I awoke the next morning, free from the emotions of the previous day, and compelled to draw upon my knowledge of elders and leadership to better understand the situation, I could see more clearly. Coming from a place of compassion instead of ego and judgment, I recognized what was happening.

My mother's identity and self-worth were bound tightly to her station as wife and mother and expert hostess. She was known for her abilities to put on a perfect meal at a perfect table in a perfect house. And the act of completing those tasks to perfection were becoming harder for her to do. She needed everything to be perfect to maintain her sense of purpose and meaning and identity. I, however, really did not care. I just wanted to get things done. Having everything perfect did not feed my need for identity and meaning as it did for her. She needed more time this year to process how to do things. I could see her stress when she could not remember how to do something. And I could see her stress when I did not do something her way, even though I thought I came to help. Her well-being was at risk. Her value was at risk. And she felt it.

Dr. Bill Thomas taught me that "the wisdom of our elders increases with the amount of honor and respect we accord them" (Thomas, personal conversation, 1998). I took that to heart the next day and found the patience to give my mother the space she needed to do things her way, no matter how long it took. I would wait for her to tell me exactly how she wanted things done and in what order she wanted them to be done. The criticisms stopped, and we had a lovely Christmas.

About 14 months later, at the age of 90, my mother was playing bridge with her friends until 11:00 at night. The next morning, she received a call from her doctor that her blood work showed that she needed to get to MD Anderson Hospital in Houston immediately, which was a 2-hour drive from her home. My brothers drove her. I flew in as quickly as I could from Denver. She was diagnosed with Acute Lymphocytic Leukemia. The prognosis was not good.

I sat in her hospital room and watched as medical professional after medical professional came in, looked at my beautiful mother lying in the bed, looked at the chart, and then looked at the door to make sure they were in the right room. Then, in an unsure voice, they would say, "Mrs. Anderson?" My mother would reply, "Yes." Then the disbelief would be verbalized. Time and time again doctors would say, "You don't look like a 90-year-old." My mother basked in that. If she did not look 90 and did not act 90, she could still have value. Then she would slather on the southern belle charm that oozed from her pores. And like everyone else that knew her, they fell in love. And they wanted to heal her.

She said she did not feel sick, and she did not look sick. This was a woman who was a survivor. She had survived the loss of a child, the loss of a grandchild, the loss of her mother and father, her husband, her sister, and brother. She had beaten breast cancer. And she convinced all of us, even her doctors, that she would beat this. So they treated her aggressively, more aggressively than they had ever treated a 90-year-old before. And she never complained. There were some days she would be at the hospital from 8:00 in the morning until well after midnight, and she never complained.

But even she could not survive this. We watched her decline. She aged 30 years in 9 months. It was like watching a sad movie. Each time I was able to visit, she was weaker. But she would not give up and she would not ask for help. She was angered by the alarm on her bed during hospital in-patient stays. I noticed a sign on her bathroom door that it was policy for everyone who was older than 65 to have a bed alarm so they would not try to get up independently. I thought to myself, "In 4 more months, I'll need a bed alarm!"

She continued aggressive treatment until the treatment became the aggressor. It was killing her. In the throes of delirium, unable to make decisions for herself any longer, my brothers and I had to make the final decision to stop aggressive treatment and keep her comfortable. I stayed with her in the palliative care unit at MD Anderson. By that time, she required 35 liters of oxygen per minute to keep her comfortable. We could not take her home. Her last words to me were, "I love you, too." She transitioned just after midnight on my 65th birthday. I think of that as her final gift to me, her way of saying goodbye.

I never had to make the decision to place my mother in a nursing home. As she was living out her final year of life surrounded by medical treatment, I was the project director for the first Green House homes in Colorado. The irony sometimes strikes me. As I was attempting to create a place where elders could live out their lives in well-being, honored for the contributions they bring to the community, my own mother was fighting to remain relevant. She was fighting to remain "young" in a world that does not honor "old." In those 7 days that I maintained vigil by her bedside, I came to understand how that belief is hurting us all.

LESSON 4
The Myth of Independence

Every successful individual knows that his or her achievement depends on a community of persons working together.

—Paul Ryan, politician

The thought of losing her independence struck fear into my mother's heart, as I am sure it also struck fear into Abigail's heart. It is one of our greatest fears of growing old. Sitting here at the age of 67 and imagining the rest of my life, that fear sometimes wraps its fingers around my throat.

I often wonder if earlier generations suffered from the same fear or are our more recent gains in longevity a driver of that fear? It is likely for Americans to live 30 years or more beyond our "working" years. We are not as likely as my grandmother's or my mother's generation to die at an early age by injury or illness. We are much more likely to develop Alzheimer's disease or a debilitating illness that could leave us vulnerable to "dependency."

The American myth is that once we reach maturity, we are all independent and our success lies in remaining independent for the rest of our lives. My mother was raised in that cowboy, bootstrap culture that deifies independence. We are all supposed to act like John Wayne, riding our horses across the desert and never needing anyone's help.

What a bunch of hooey! The fact is that we are not independent. In his book, *What Are Old People For? How Elders Will Save the World*, Dr. Bill Thomas speaks to this myth (2004, p. 241):

Myth: To be dependent is to rely on others for the most basic necessities of life.

Reality: To be dependent is to be human. We all rely on others for the necessities of life. The form this reliance takes adds to or detracts from our well-being.

Think about something that you do independently, other than through your autonomic nervous system functions, which regulate the function of internal organs and are involuntary. You do not have control over these; your nervous system does. Try holding your breath until you die. You cannot do it. As soon as you pass out, your nervous system will breathe for you. It is not a great idea to test out that hypothesis. Trust me on this one.

Other than involuntary functions, what else do you do independently? Be careful. You know this is a trick question; the answer is nothing. Everything we do for the necessities of life, we do while relying on others. That is, unless you are John Wayne.

I do not grow all of my own food. I go to the grocery store. I did not build my own shelter. I walk into my house, flip a switch, and, voilà, electricity. I turn on the faucet and have water. That water drains somewhere, but I did not build the sewer or make the pipes. You get my drift. In this modern day, we all rely on others for our most basic necessities of life. Actually, we always have.

None of us is truly independent. We are and always have been interdependent. Emily Wyman and Esther Herrmann remind us about the evolution of human cooperation: "As compared with other primates, human beings are inordinately cooperative, especially with nonrelatives" (Tomasello, Melis, Tennie, Wyman, & Hermann, 2012, p. 673).

Our very success as humans depends upon how well we have cooperated with others. Know that. Dr. Thomas's quote reminds us that the form of this reliance on others can enhance or detract from our well-being.

When that reliance is cooperative and supportive, it enhances our well-being. When we can continue to give to others in some way, our well-being is supported. When we continue to have autonomy over our lives and meaning in our lives, then this interdependence helps us. It is only when our partners in care remove our autonomy, strip our lives of meaning, or deny us the opportunity to give as well as receive that our reliance on others becomes detrimental to our well-being.

When I was trying to be in charge in my mother's kitchen or do for her instead of letting her direct me, her wisdom and her well-being were diminished. And in that process, I diminished my own well-being. Understanding this, finally, I was able to support her by honoring her and her autonomy. And my life was easier because I changed. If only I could have figured that out at age 13 instead of 63. I rest easy knowing that for the remainder of her life after that Christmas, I supported her decisions, even if they were not the decisions I would make for myself.

It is important for person-centered leaders to understand how this myth of independence affects our elders. It is vital to our elders' well-being that we create caring communities where they can continue to direct their own lives, where they can continue to find ways to give back, and where they can live embraced in the arms of interdependence and without the threat of dependence.

It is also important for person-centered leaders to recognize how this myth of independence is hurting our staff. Because of the myth, staff members believe they can be successful by themselves. Day after day, in thousands of care communities in this country, hundreds of thousands of elder caregivers are running around like chickens with their heads cut off, trying to complete all of their tasks. Rarely will they ask for help, unless there is some penalty threatened (e.g., if they do not use two people for the Hoyer lift). Managers will not ask for help from each other. Hands-on staff do a little better just because some of their tasks are impossible to do alone. But for the most part, we believe that we are independent. In fact, much of the conflict among nursing home employees happens because we do depend on each other for success. And when the "night shift left it" or the "social worker didn't complete her MDS," there will be trouble. No wonder we have a bunch of people acting like martyrs (e.g., "No one works as hard as I do"). No wonder we have people rushing madly about, bemoaning that there is not enough time. We have bought into the myth. It is ingrained in our culture. But you cannot be successful by yourself.

UBUNTU

This is not the culture in other parts of the world. Rayne Stroebel, my colleague and Eden Regional Coordinator for South Africa, spoke at the 2014 Eden International Conference, during which he introduced the largely American audience to the concept of Ubuntu (pronounced *u-boon-tu*), an ancient African philosophy and way of life. The word has many meanings, but the Archbishop Desmond Tutu defines Ubuntu as "I am who I am because we are who we are." With Ubuntu, the belief is that we are all connected by a universal bond across all humanity. Talk about interdependence!

The Archbishop explains,

> We believe that a person is a person through another person, that my humanity is caught up, bound up, inextricably, with yours. When I dehumanize you, I inexorably dehumanize myself. The solitary human is a contradiction in terms and therefore you seek to work for the common good because your humanity comes into its own in belonging. (Tutu Foundation, 2016)

The following story made the rounds through social media in 2012 and speaks to this culture of Ubuntu:

> An anthropologist studying the habits and customs of an African tribe found himself surrounded by children most days. So he decided to play a little game with them. He managed to get candy from the nearest town and put it all in a decorated basket at the foot of a tree.
>
> Then he called the children and suggested they play the game. When the anthropologist said "now," the children had to run to the tree; the first one to get there could have all the candy to him/herself.
>
> So the children all lined up, waiting for the signal. When the anthropologist said "now," all of the children took each other by the hand ran together towards the tree. They all arrived at the same time, divided up the candy, sat down, and began to happily munch away.
>
> The anthropologist went over to them and asked why they had all run together when any one of them could have had the candy all to themselves.
>
> The children responded: "Ubuntu. How could any one of us be happy if all the others were sad?

Imagine for a moment that you were able to create that kind of culture in your care community. Do you think you would have any problems finding people who wanted to live or work there?

Person-centered leaders dispel the myth of independence and replace it with the truth of a caring community, of interdependence. They recognize the leadership imperative that comes with their positions: to narrow the gap between the way things are and the way they ought to be. The lessons in Chapter 2 teach us more about creating caring communities where everyone, including the leaders, can be happy.

CHAPTER 2

How It Ought To Be

Three Stories & One Myth

The Mystery of Roseto

The new currency won't be intellectual capital. It will be social capital, the collective value of whom we know and what we'll do for each other. When social connections are strong and numerous, there is more trust, reciprocity, information flow, collective action, happiness, and, by the way, greater wealth.

—James Kouzes, Chairman Emeritus of Tom Peters Company

Roseto, Pennsylvania, was an example of a truly caring community. Everyone who was lucky enough to live in Roseto in the 1950s and 1960s benefitted from the well-being that can be created through social capital. What healthcare providers learned from this community must not be ignored, for it proves the value of living, working, and aging in communities rather than institutions.

The small community of Roseto in east-central Pennsylvania was founded in the late-nineteenth century by a group of immigrants from a town of the same name in Italy. Stewart Wolf was a physician and professor in Oklahoma who grew up near Roseto and continued to return to the area during the summers. During one of these summers in the late 1950s, he was invited to speak at a local medical society meeting. There he ran into a colleague, another physician who had practiced in the area for 17 years. That colleague happened to mention to Wolf something about his practice that Wolf felt was very odd: he had never treated anyone from Roseto under the age of 65 with heart disease.

This was the late 1950s, before the advent of cholesterol lowering drugs and stents. The effects of smoking, cholesterol, high blood pressure, and obesity on the development of heart disease were unknown. Following a heart attack, there were limited treatments for the damage suffered to the heart, so it was not uncommon for Americans to die of heart attacks in their 50s or 60s. But not, it seemed, if you lived in Roseto.

This intrigued Wolf, so he and another researcher from Oklahoma, John Bruhn, decided to make a trip to Roseto to see what they could find. Wolf, Bruhn, and their team of researchers conducted an extensive study to compare the medical histories of a large sample of Rosetans and members of two surrounding communities. The results were stunning. At a time when heart attacks in the United States were on the rise, Wolf and Bruhn found that:

- No one in Roseto younger than 55 had died of a heart attack or showed any signs of heart disease.

- For men older than 65, the death rate from heart disease was half that of the United States as a whole.

- There was no suicide, alcoholism, or drug addiction, and very little crime.

- People were dying of old age. That's it.

When confronted with these statistics, Wolf and Bruhn first thought about diet and lifestyle. Had the Rosetans continued the old world ways of preparing food and eating? No. In fact, they found that 41% of their calories came from fat. The Rosetans smoked heavily and did not exercise. Many were struggling with obesity. They had all of the indicators for heart disease, but no symptoms. This led Wolf and Bruhn to consider genetic makeup. They found relatives of the Rosetans who lived in other parts of the country, but these relatives had average health. Next, they pondered whether it might be something in the environment. But when they studied health statistics from the two closest towns, they found death rates to be three times those of Roseto.

Why didn't the Rosetans have heart disease? What was going on in Roseto?

These puzzling results led Wolf and Bruhn to conduct an extensive 15-year study of Roseto that is detailed in their book, *The Roseto Study: An Anatomy of Health,* published in 1979. What they found may surprise you as much as it surprised the medical community. Wolf and Bruhn found that Rosetans had created a "powerful, protective social structure that insulated them from the pressures of the modern world."

There were extended family clans. Three generations lived under one roof. Grandparents commanded great respect in Roseto and maintained their authority throughout life. The Rosetans sat on their porches, walked down the streets of the community, and talked to each other daily. They shared meals together. They worked together, played together, and cared for each other. There were 22 separate civic organizations in a town of just under 2,000. The Rosetans had created an egalitarian ethos in which the wealthy restrained their inclination toward material possession, resulting in a "classless" society.

The Rosetans had created a community not of blood kin, but of affection toward one another. The close social connections that were formed protected them from stress, poor dietary habits and lifestyles, and the devastation of a hierarchical society. That social capital even protected them from heart disease.

This research completely changed the way healthcare providers looked at the health of individuals. No longer could they just look at the person, his or her genetics and lifestyle choices. What this research and much further research have shown is that health must be examined in the context of overall culture (Bruhn & Wolf, 1979).

Social capital can be defined as "the network of social connections that exists between people, and their shared values and norms of behavior, which enable and encourage mutually advantageous social cooperation" (Dictionary.com). Although the term *social capital* has been around for decades, it has become more popularized though the work of Robert Putnam (2000) in his groundbreaking book, *Bowling Alone: The Collapse and Revival of American Community*. In this book, Putnam argues that although Americans have significantly increased their financial capital, they have lost social capital in the process, including all of the benefits that social capital brings to well-being. According to Putnam, "A society characterized by generalized reciprocity is more efficient than a distrustful society, for the same reason that money is more efficient than barter. If we don't have to balance every exchange instantly, we can get more accomplished" (Putnam, 2000, p. 21).

Reciprocity is the outcome of a high-trust environment. High trust only comes from strong relationships and a deep knowing. In this way, social capital can be the lubricant for a higher-functioning organization.

Many empirical studies have been conducted to determine the impact of social capital on not just our health, but also on our overall well-being and the well-being of our organizations. As James Kouzes expresses in the quote at the beginning of this lesson, the "new currency will be . . . social capital."

If we are to call ourselves healthcare providers, we must learn the lessons that Roseto offers us about the impact and value of social capital and of a caring community on human health, not just that of our residents, but also of our employees and ourselves.

Formal leaders in the new culture of care must do everything they can to replicate the kind of caring community that employs social capital as a driving force of the well-being of all.

LESSON 6
Lessons from Roscoe Elementary School

Without a sense of caring, there can be no sense of community.

—Anthony J. D'Angelo, founder of Collegiate EmPowerment

Roscoe Elementary School was as unlikely a candidate for deep cultural transformation as might be found. Located 16 miles from downtown Los Angeles, Roscoe Elementary is part of the second-largest school district in the United States. The school is adjacent to an industrial and commercial area and serves a neighborhood of apartment buildings and tiny, single-family homes. The majority of the residents are blue collar workers and unskilled laborers, mostly immigrants from Latin America, Southeast Asia, and the Middle East. The area served is made up of a very transient, impoverished, multicultural, and multilingual population. The odds were greatly against Roscoe Elementary ever cultivating a caring community as was found in Roseto, Pennsylvania. Yet, through wise leadership, redesigned school structures, an altered definition of success, and a focus on building relationships, Roscoe Elementary beat the odds.

Roscoe Elementary is not a nursing home, but their success in community building can be easily translated to the long-term care arena. We have much to learn from Roscoe's journey of transformation as we undertake or continue on our own journeys toward cultivating caring communities.

A study conducted at Roscoe during one school year in the mid-1990s examined how this urban elementary school manifested characteristics of a caring community. The study revealed three central themes that are consistent with creating a caring community:

1. "A climate of mutual trust and respect pervaded the entire institution." (Kratzer, 1997, p. 351)

The researchers found that: *"Creating a climate of trust and respect begins with leadership. At Roscoe, administrators consciously modeled attitudes of respect and trust toward all stakeholders"* (Kratzer, 1997, p. 352).

With communities following the institutional model, I find a lack of trust is fostered by administrators who blame families, surveyors, corporate staff, and even plaintiffs' attorneys for their problems. Department managers hunker down in their own department silos and take pot shots at each other, or they malign an entire generation of workers with statements such as, "There is just no work ethic anymore." Finger-pointing and blaming are the norm, not the exception. Trust and respect fly out the window in this type of environment. A person-centered culture begins not with big changes, but with changing our most basic behaviors in how we treat each other. Formal leaders must set the bar high and demand respect of everyone by everyone at all times.

2. "There were fluid boundaries around an ethic of caring." (Kratzer, 1997, p. 345)

The researchers found that: *"Formal roles and structures at Roscoe were less critical and influential than were relationships and informal interactions. An attitude of helping and caring extended beyond the professional level"* (Kratzer, 1997, p. 354).

Boundaries too often divide and separate. We like them because they offer some sense of structure. When boundaries become fluid, however, they can help break down divisions between hierarchies, roles, and functions to create a new kind of organization.

This is not to suggest that you do away with formal boundaries. I am just suggesting that when you create a caring community, those boundaries become less important. They become flexible. When leaders focus on the process of growing relationships among all stakeholders, those boundary lines are blurred. It may not be in my job description to mop the spill on the floor, but I do it because I have a relationship with the housekeeper and I am willing to help her. I also do not want anyone to slip and fall waiting for the spill to be cleaned. I behave the way any caring person would behave in a community.

3. "A collective and individual sense of ownership and responsibility permeated the community at all levels." (Kratzer, 1997, p. 356)

The researchers found that: *"Individual and collective ownership and responsibility for the well-being of the community and its members permeated the community at all levels at Roscoe. There was a deep recognition of the need to work together toward the common good"* (Kratzer, 1997, p. 348).

This is what I call "universal accountability." In the institutional model, one or more formal leaders make a decision to do something differently, then they go out and try to "sell" that idea to the stakeholders. They try to get "buy-in." This is rarely effective. In a human community, each stakeholder has a voice in shared decision making. If you want a caring community, you need ownership, not buy-in, from all members. Ownership comes only with a voice in shaping the plan.

These three central elements combined to create a *"strong sense of caring at Roscoe that was palpable even to visitors first visiting the school, and continued to be evident over time"* (Kratzer, 1997, p. 351).

The lessons for long-term care leaders can be found in how this school was able to make and sustain this kind of authentic community. The text boxes that follow are my suggestions for replicating the results at Roscoe Elementary.

Creating a Climate of Mutual Trust and Respect in Your Care Community

- Help each person become well known. Cultivate strong relationships throughout the care community. In the institutional model, people are not known and relationships do not matter.

- Foster a mutual understanding of the inherent worth of each person (yes, even the worth of the state surveyors).

- Create shared values and bind those values to common goals. Members of the community share values, especially the idea that they belong to a common entity that supersedes the interests of individual members. Set standards of conduct (See Lesson 30).

- Create a climate of tolerance toward differing opinions. (Stop saying, "That will never work" or "We tried that already.") Intentionally hire independent-minded employees, encourage minority viewpoints, and show that you are open to new ideas and suggestions.

- Use communication tools, such as learning circles and huddles, daily (see Lesson 30). The more community members share, or at least understand and tolerate, each other's values and attitudes, the stronger their community will be.

- Celebrate and honor diversity. Set aside a day or month for each ethnicity or nationality in your community to share their culture, including stories, dress, food, and music.

- Encourage and welcome concerns from residents and families, and respond to those concerns quickly. Re-educate staff to view complaints as gifts.

- Engage all stakeholders in the decision making and governance of the community.

- Become vulnerable. Admit your mistakes and ask staff to help you conduct a root-cause analysis of your mistake.

- Invite staff to help you grow by telling you if you ever do anything to hurt their feelings.

- Share decision making with other stakeholders.

Creating an Ethic of Caring in Your Community

- Grow neighborhood or household teams. Encourage collaboration and congeniality between departments, shifts, managers, and staff.
- Cross-train staff and blend roles.
- Encourage other members of the community to help each other out in times of personal crisis (e.g., bringing meals to a co-worker's house in times of emergency; ensure managers work in the dining room during meals; cover for an employee so that she or he can go home to take care of a sick child).
- Refrain from reprimanding people who call in sick. Ask how you can help.
- Share home-cooked food. Plan social gatherings together.
- Create rituals to welcome new members to the community, both residents and staff.
- Teach conflict resolution and manage conflict so that it is not left to fester.
- Create opportunities for employees, residents, and families to share their own passions and skills by leading team meetings, teaching, or mentoring.
- Welcome families and use the community's resources to help them in times of need. Involve families in the governance of the community.
- Promote and encourage a sense of fun and play in the community.
- Encourage all managers to conduct one activity per month in the community, bringing their passions to work.

Creating a Collective and Individual Sense of Ownership and Responsibility in Your Care Community

- Hold daily community meetings with residents and staff.
- Engage all stakeholders in creating new mission and vision statements, and sharing in the direction of the community by introducing new ideas.
- Encourage administrators and managers to become facilitators and coaches who empower neighborhood teams. Engage in shared decision making and collaborative problem solving.
- Give staff opportunities to explore new ways of doing things. Remove the fear of failure.
- Create a culture that believes everyone is responsible for all residents, not just those in a neighborhood or only hands-on staff. Model that behavior.
- Make call lights stop lights; no one can pass by one. Phones are emergency sirens. Train everyone on how to answer a phone so that no one passes a ringing or flashing light.
- Encourage everyone to participate in caring for the community. Give neighborhood teams, residents, and families opportunities to design the look of their neighborhood, within parameters, and assist in transforming the look.
- Clean up the home to create a safe and orderly environment. Keep cleaning supplies and equipment available in the neighborhoods and expect everyone to participate in keeping the home clean, instead of waiting on the housekeeping staff. Have a Spring Cleaning Day, and invite everyone to kick off the new initiative.
- Come up with a community song and slogan. Provide staff and families community t-shirts with the slogan.
- Redefine success beyond current measures of census, lack of deficiencies, and quality of care. Raise expectations to include the quality of life and well-being of all stakeholders.
- Include members of all stakeholder groups in the interviewing and hiring process.
- Create a well-being committee of all stakeholders and have them come up with ideas for improving the well-being of residents and staff.

LESSON 7
Saint Lucia

We must accept finite disappointment, but never lose infinite hope.

—Martin Luther King, Jr., civil rights activist and minister

SAINT LUCIA, 2007

Through my work with The Eden Alternative, I came to know some great administrator leaders. None of them had a bigger heart or more courage than Dorene Spies, who ran a home in Nebraska that was owned by an order of nuns. She called them her "nunny-bunnies."

This order of nuns also operated homes in the Caribbean, including one in the capital city of Saint Lucia, Castries. Although Saint Lucia has become a popular tourist destination, almost a third of the country's population still lives in poverty. The home was located in a part of Castries where that poverty was direst. In 2006, at the request of the Sisters, Dorene took a group of people to Saint Lucia to help the home. She was returning again the next year and asked me to join them.

We brought suitcases full of items the home would need, everything from linens and towels to toothbrushes, medical supplies, and clothing for the elders. We landed in Castries at 9:00 p.m. We prayed we would make it through customs with our "stash." As we stepped off the plane, we were hit with a wall of heat and humidity that is difficult to describe. And I am from Texas. We would continue to experience this same heat index throughout our stay, for we were not headed to a resort with a cool sea breeze and drinks with umbrellas in them. We were headed into a part of town where the police do not venture into after dark.

I have seen some poverty in my time, but nothing like this. The hillside beyond the nursing home gates was littered with homemade huts made of tin and cardboard, stacked one on top of the other without enough space between them for even a gentle breeze from the sea to penetrate. At one point during our stay, I asked one of the nuns who oversaw the nursing home why they did not have a garden. She explained that the plants would be stolen before they could produce a harvest.

A fence surrounded the property, but this did not deter the thieves. Every night, they came into the compound. They engineered elaborate devices out of tree branches and thorny plants that they would use to reach through the louvered windows, trying to grab items we left too close to the windows. They climbed the walls of the convent and broke into the nuns' sleeping quarters, stealing away with anything they could gather. One of the first tasks we undertook was to fix the iron gate the thieves had rigged for ease of entry.

These were not bad people; they were desperate people who were steeped in dire poverty, stranded on an island with no hope of finding a means of making a living. They were only trying to survive.

The nursing home was run by a 70-year-old nun named Sister Amadeus. She stood all of 5 feet tall, with a round face, glasses, and a full habit replete with dark support hose and those bulky "nun shoes." While I was shedding clothes as quickly as I could in the oppressive heat of Saint Lucia, this amazing woman did not ever break a sweat. And she had plenty to sweat about.

She ran a nursing home of about 60 people. Only three of the elders who lived there could contribute any funds toward their care. The rest relied heavily upon a quarterly stipend from the government. On our first full day on the island, the government was more than 30 days late with the payment. That night, the elders who lived in this home had as their evening meal three small slices of French bread, the size of a plum, with peanut butter.

The home was two stories with a balcony that ran the length of the second story, where elders spent much of their day, trying to catch a whisper of an ocean breeze. Each morning as we passed by and asked how they were, they replied, "Nothing to complain." They had nothing, yet they had "nothing to complain."

The elders lived in two large rooms, the women upstairs and the men downstairs. Their beds, lined up on each side of the room, were ancient and rusted from the sea air. The walls were stained and dirty, a lifeless hospital green that had faded and mildewed throughout the years. Many of the elders lived with diabetes, exacerbated by a diet low in protein and high in carbohydrates.

We spent the first few days hauling out broken equipment, outdated and tattered supplies, and threadbare and dry-rotted linens. Every closet and storage area was jammed full of useless items. It seems when one lives with scarcity, one never throws anything away. We found medications from 1950 and equipment that would never be usable again jammed into every available space. We brought new supplies, linens, equipment, and clothing to replace the items we were throwing away.

We painted the walls with bright colors. The women who worked in the laundry wore these beautiful, bright, lime-green suits to work every day, and every day they worked in oppressive heat with one small washing machine that was on its last leg. They hung the clothes to dry on strings of telephone wire they had rigged together. We brought a new washing machine and built new areas for drying the clothes.

Because the government had not paid their quarterly stipend to the home, the staff had not been paid for over a month. The home was receiving cut-off notices from the water and electric companies for having been delinquent for several months.

As I took in the state of affairs in this home, I could feel an uneasiness stirring in me. I was becoming more and more agitated at the injustice of it all. I did not understand why I was brought there to witness this injustice. I did not really have anything to contribute. I was not a nurse or a doctor. Sure, I could paint and clean and haul trash, but what real difference was I making? I was a nursing home administrator. I was used to solving problems, but this problem was too big for me to solve. My agitation grew.

One day, the Minister of Health for Saint Lucia was slated to tour all of the nursing homes on the island. I asked Sister Amadeus if I could meet with her. I was prepared to give the Minister of Health a piece of my mind. Sister Amadeus told me I could not meet with her. When I asked her why, she said, "You will only anger her, and I don't need her anger." Wise woman.

That day, as Sister Amadeus stood outside awaiting the Minister of Health's visit, the man from the water company came to cut off the water. Sister Amadeus spoke to him and said, "Please do not cut off the water, these people will die." The man just replied, "I'm sorry, Sister, but it is my job." "Yes, you are right," the Sister replied, "You must do your job. But after you cut off the water, I want you to go into town and bring us a truck with water so these people do not die." The man left without cutting off the water.

My agitation was growing the longer Sister Amadeus waited for the Minister of Health. I was trying to keep busy, but every time I saw another injustice, I got angrier and angrier. Dorene and I were walking past an elder on the porch, when I noticed an ant crawling across her foot. I bent down to swipe the ant off her foot and saw several more crawling on her. We always carried bottles of water with us everywhere to try to keep from getting dehydrated, so I opened my bottle and poured a little water on her foot to wash the ants off. When I did that, her toes spread and I saw she had a wound between her toes. As I bent to look closer, dozens of ants poured out of the wound onto the top of her foot. I kept pouring water, trying to wash them away. At the same time, I called to Dorene to get a nurse. This woman was infested with ants! I kept pouring water, desperately trying to get the ants off of her, but more and more kept coming out of this wound. Finally, one of their nurses came running downstairs. I looked up and saw what she had in her hand. It was a can of ant killer! I screamed, "No! Dorene, get one of our nurses."

By the time our nurse arrived, I had managed to get the ants off the elder. The nurse took her away to attend to her wound. I lost it then. I went into full administrator mode. I needed information so I could problem solve. I screamed in my head, "Why am I here?" I screamed at Dorene, "What the Hell is going on here? I need to see the budget!" Dorene looked at me like I had lost my mind, which was a pretty accurate assessment at that point. She smiled and said, "I don't think there is a budget." I said, "What do you mean? How can they run a nursing home without a budget?" She replied, "I can ask, but I doubt they have one."

A short time later, we were sitting in the small office when Sister Amadeus came in carrying an old leather ledger. She placed it in front of me and nodded. I opened it to discover page after page of entries written in a beautiful small script. I scoured the pages of debits and credits. You can guess which had more entries. It did not take me long to realize that this home was losing about $100,000EC a year. At that time, the exchange rate between the U.S. dollar and the East Caribbean Dollar was about $1US to $2.50EC.

The Minister of Health never came that day. She was too busy visiting the private homes on the island. And I am sure she was embarrassed and ashamed (at least I hope she was) that her government had not paid this home their quarterly stipend. The situation was grave. Both the electric company and water company were on the verge of discontinuing services. The staff had not been paid in over a month, yet they still came to work. Their husbands even went fishing and brought fish for the elders to eat. They could not grow a garden or even enjoy the mangoes from the trees, as thieves would come in the night and steal them. Each day, a white male priest with starched and pressed vestments would come to the home to deliver mass. The nuns would faithfully attend. Then the priest would return to his condo, leaving the nuns to do the best they could in a place where police were afraid to come during the night. They were on their own.

As I looked at the ledger and looked up at this amazing 70-year-old woman, I lost hope. I fell into deep despair. I just shook my head and said to her, "How do you do it?" She replied, "By the grace of God." I know the sun must have addled my brain, because I then said (to a nun), "God! Where is God? Show me God!" Without missing a beat, she looked me straight in the eye and said, "He sent you," three small words spoken softly without a shred of doubt.

It was as if she had thrown a bucket of ice water in my face, which might have been what I deserved at that moment. But all she said was, "He sent you." Now, I do not care if you are a religious person or not. I do not care whether you are a believer or not. If you had been in my place at that moment in time, you may have heard what I heard, which was, "Stop whining and do something! You are here for a week; this is my life."

So I said, "I need a phone. Get me a phone."

I placed a call to The Eden Alternative home office and told my staff that I was going to fax a letter that I wanted them to send to everyone in our database. This was a crisis. Elders were going to die if we did not do something quickly. I then wrote a plea to our "tribe." I told them about these elders who had nothing and who had nothing to complain. I told them about the staff who came to work even though they had not been paid. I asked for their help. And the help came. From around the Eden world, the dollars poured into the Eden office. Within 24 hours, we had raised almost $10,000US.

The money was wired to the Western Union Office in Castries, Saint Lucia. Now the question became how to get $10,000US ($25,000 in their currency) safely to the convent. Fortunately for us, a young man was visiting the home who had grown up in Castries but had traveled extensively and gone to school in the United States. And he had a car. So, Sister Amadeus and I drove with him to the bank. The plan was for him to let us out, then circle the block while we collected the money. Sister Amadeus and I zipped into the bank. She had a large, leather satchel that we filled with the cash. With it pressed firmly across her bosom, we waited until we saw the car turn the corner. Then, like an odd couple Bonnie and Clyde, we ran out the door and jumped in the car.

When we arrived back at the convent, Sister Amadeus took the money up to her quarters. I wondered how she would dole it out. Would she pay the water and electric bills? It was not enough to get them out of debt, and it certainly was not enough to ensure their sustainability. My questions were answered a short time later, when I saw a line of staff going up to the nuns' quarters. She was paying her staff first. Yes!

That day, I learned from a great leader. That day, I learned about the power of hope in the midst of the direst of circumstances. That day, a diminutive elder nun stood up for what was right. In the midst of finite disappointment, she never for a moment lost "infinite hope." She challenged all of us to do the same. Great leaders deal in hope, not despair or fear.

The next day we threw a party for the elders and staff. I invited Sister Amadeus to dance with me and darned if she did not take me up on it! Her staff was amazed. They laughed and laughed, and we danced and danced. Dorene continues to take mission groups to Saint Lucia each year to help the home. That's what great leaders do.

LESSON 8
The Turnover Myth

Managers tend to blame their turnover problems on everything under the sun, while ignoring the crux of the matter: people don't leave jobs; they leave managers.

—Travis Bradberry, author

Research now shows us the importance of leadership in the success of our care communities. Ask yourself if you agree or disagree with the following statement: Understaffing and inconsistent staffing are associated with poor quality nursing home care (Kayser-Jones, Schell, & Kramer, 1997; Kramer & Fish, 2001).

Has that been your experience? Can you deliver quality care without sufficient staff? Can you deliver the highest quality care if you are moving staff all over and not providing consistent assignment? Care communities, are not high tech. The quality of the services care communities deliver is dependent upon having sufficient, well-trained, compassionate, caring, hands-on staff. Do you agree? If so, do you agree with this next statement: *Turnover can be a major financial and time drain on a care community.*

Do you actually know the financial cost of your turnover? Have you analyzed your turnover and completed a root cause analysis of it? Do you have an action plan in place to address staff stability?

Do you analyze your food costs? Your supply costs? Of course you do. You do that because you can control those costs. In my experience, I have found very few formal leaders in care communities who spend as much time analyzing their labor costs as they do their food costs. And if they do, they rarely include the cost of turnover. Analysis should include the cost of staff time to recruit, interview and hire, and orient and train.

If labor costs are our largest cost center, by far, why are we not paying more attention to it?

Maybe because we do not think we can control turnover. That is the turnover myth.

Do you agree with this last statement: *The increase in care needs of an aging population will create even more competition for staff positions.*

The challenges we have been experiencing with staff stability are likely to get worse, as there is more competition in our labor market.

So what does staff stability have to do with leadership? In a word, everything. I am convinced, and at some point I hope you will be as well, that it is entirely possible through leadership to create a place where people want to live and work. I am convinced that the path to improving staff stability is waiting for each of us to discover.

In 2001, Susan Eaton, assistant professor of public policy at Harvard who had studied long-term care settings for more than 20 years, was contracted by the Centers for Medicare & Medicaid Services (CMS) to conduct a study of the variation of turnover among nursing staff (nurses and certified nursing assistants [CNAs]) within a single labor market. The study was commissioned to address two important questions:

1. Why does turnover among nursing staff vary widely in long-term care institutions, even among facilities located close together?

2. What difference can management practices make in helping to understand the mechanisms associated with either high or low turnover?

The research was conducted during the spring and summer of 2001 in nine long-term care facilities in four labor markets in three states: California, Kansas, and Wisconsin. The research was done as part of a federally mandated study on the appropriateness of establishing minimum nursing staff in nursing facilities. Researchers selected facilities in the top and bottom quadrant of turnover, within the same labor market, and within each state. The idea was to compare "apples to apples." Why were some workers likely to stay in jobs at a nursing facility in a local area when similar workers were likely to leave another nursing facility down the street? The study was designed to delve deeply into the reasons for turnover in a market where CNAs and nursing staff had real choices about where to work.

Eaton's study uncovered some typical explanations for high turnover among direct care staff in nursing homes:

- "These are marginal job seekers who cannot keep a job, come to work regularly, or perform reliably."

- "These are often poor workers, many single parents, who have little support at home."

- "These workers do not have a good work ethic as contrasted with workers of the previous generation."

- "These are typically low-wage workers who have lower job commitment and attachment in general."

- "These are often immigrant workers who may have trouble with work status, the law, school, or relatives who live distances away."

- "These are workers for whom serious economic and life problems are only one paycheck away, often without health insurance, savings, or retirement. They are not likely to be stable, committed workers as life difficulties can prevent them from attending work regularly."

Do you hold any of those beliefs?

I am certain there are examples of each of these explanations in the long-term care workforce. Eaton claims, however, that the varying turnover rate among homes in the same area makes some of these broad explanations of limited use. She found, for example, that managers in the high-turnover homes tended to see turnover as inevitable. Most of these homes had in excess of 100% turnover annually. Managers in the low-turnover homes knew they had relatively low turnover, 30% or less, but were troubled by their turnover. The national average for turnover in all industries (excluding layoffs) ranges between 10% and 20%.

Eaton's study identified many specific managerial practices that differed between low-turnover and high-turnover homes. Five of these practices stand out:

1. "High quality leadership and management offering recognition, meaning, and feedback, as well as the opportunity to

see one's work as valued and valuable; managers who built on the intrinsic motivation of workers in this field."

2. "An organizational culture, communicated by managers, families, supervisors, and the nurses, of valuing and respecting nursing caregivers themselves as well as the residents."

3. "Basic positive or 'high performance' Human Resource Policies, including wages and benefits, but also in the areas of soft skills and flexibility, training and career ladders, scheduling, realistic job previews."

4. "Thoughtful and effective motivational work organization and care practices. Good systems, good organization, easy access to equipment and supplies."

5. "Adequate staffing ratios and resources for giving high quality of care."

How many of these practices do you, as leaders in an organization, have control over? Is staff turnover inevitable, or is it within your purview to affect?

Eaton's research is titled "What a difference management makes!" Good sound management practices are critical to the success of our communities. But I am going to go one more step and say, "What a difference leadership makes!"

Great leaders who understand the benefits of good management practices also know the importance of driving leadership deep within their communities, so that everyone is acting as a leader.

I want you to imagine a community in which turnover is minimal because people want to work there. I want you to imagine a community in which you have a waiting list for staff positions. I want you to imagine a world in which the people you are coaching reach their maximum potential because of your efforts. That world is possible through your leadership.

If we are going to learn the lessons of Roseto, Roscoe Elementary School, and Saint Lucia as well as debunk the turnover myth, then we must explore the concept of person-centered leadership.

Leadership is not something that is easily defined. If I were to ask 100 people to tell me the definition of leadership, I would probably get 100 different answers. Sure, many of those answers would have some commonalities, but to nail down just one definition of leadership is challenging, at best.

Socrates had a method he would often use to define something that was difficult to define. He would have a dialog with others about its opposite. By defining what it is not, the definition of what it is became clearer. Let us try that by defining what the institutional model taught us about leadership, because that is about as opposite from person-centered leadership as you can get.

The institutional model gave us one picture of leadership, and it goes something like this:

- You have to have a title to be a leader; no one else is expected to be a leader.

- Leaders hold all of the decision-making authority and have the right to filter down this authority as they see fit without ever truly empowering others.

- Formal leaders hold all of the information and dole it out on a "need to know" basis; unless you hold a title, you have little need to know.

- It is the job of formal leaders to hold others accountable, so they chase behind people like sheepherder dogs, nipping at their heels, trying to keep everyone in line.

- Because leaders hold all of the authority, they also hold all of the accountability. So these few very committed, caring, and tireless people work themselves until they burn out.

- Accountability is weaponized. Leaders use fear as a motivating factor because they believe it is the only way to hold people accountable. This creates an "us and them" context where the divide between management and staff or between corporate staff and facility staff is wider than the Grand Canyon.

- Managers tend to judge their employees based upon attendance and timely task completion. Because there are few people who want to work in this type of environment, they tend to settle for less than the best in their employees. They fear not having enough staff, and allow bad behaviors in staff to go on forever. Managers follow the "science" of management theory, but not even the most current management theory. Many formal leaders in the institutional model are still stuck in the beginning of the last century in applying a scientific management style.

Frederick Taylor developed the "scientific management theory," which espoused this careful specification and measurement of all organizational tasks. Tasks were standardized as much as possible. Workers were rewarded and punished based on managers' inspections of their work. This approach appeared to work well for organizations with assembly lines and other mechanistic, routinized activities.

Businesses, however, gave up that style of management more than 50 years ago because it did not work. It was supposed to have been an efficiency model, but it was anything but efficient. They began to recognize that they needed to involve the workers in the design, evaluation, and improvement of the work. So they changed.

Except in healthcare, which is still stuck in the early 20th century in management theory.

Out of the ashes of the institutional model, however, a new kind of leadership is emerging. This leadership is an art, not a science. But like any art, it relies upon the science of leadership to inform and elevate it to its highest level. Some tenets of this new thinking include the following:

- Person-centered leaders believe that leadership is a behavior, not a position. All of us will at times be called to act as leaders, not just those of us with formal titles. Titles do not buy you anything but a little bit of time. What you do with that time will determine if you are a leader of people or not. There are many people in positions of formal authority in this world who are not acting like leaders. When that happens, people get hurt. A person-centered leader recognizes the potential in each person, then grows herself so that she can help others to grow. She understands that when everyone in her organization is acting as a leader, there is no problem too big or challenge too great to meet.

- Formal leaders in a person-centered care model share decision-making authority throughout their community. They recognize that wisdom is not found in only one person's head. They also understand the latest research on human motivation, which reveals autonomy as one of the most powerful intrinsic human motivators. We are all born with a need for autonomy. Planning, evaluating, and directing one's own work life through empowerment helps meet this basic human need.

- Person-centered leaders understand that information is power and that empowered teams need all of the information available in order to make good decisions. These leaders are transparent and freely share information with everyone in the organization. This builds trust and understanding and narrows the gap between management and staff.

- Person-centered leaders understand their job is to create a context in which everyone can reach their highest potential. That involves creating a context of universal accountability, where everyone is accountable, rather than hierarchical accountability, where only a few are accountable.

- Person-centered leaders redefine accountability as growth. They support universal accountability in which people care for each other by helping each other to grow. They do not need to use fear or threats; they have other ways of influencing behavior.

- Person-centered leaders have the highest expectations of their employees, and they help them to meet those expectations by clearly communicating with each person about expectations and their progress in meeting those expectations. They model the behaviors they want to see in their employees.

- Person-centered leaders use the latest evidence-based science to inform the art of their leadership. They understand that they have to grow themselves before they can expect others to grow. They understand that they create the context in which all behavior occurs.

I want to offer you a definition of person-centered leadership based on these tenets and new behaviors: *Person-centered leadership is the ability to create a context in which each person has the potential to be the best he or she can be for the world.*

There is a leadership imperative built into the person-centered model that is not present in the institutional model. It is relatively easy to create and sustain an institution; maybe not satisfying or meaningful, but relatively easy.

To create and sustain an institution, one need only develop some policies and procedures, some disciplinary policies, some clearly defined job descriptions, and demarcated boundary lines. Then sit back and wait for people to break those policies or cross those boundaries, and punish them when they do. And while punishing them, make sure you threaten them with even greater punishment should they do it again. Then you just treat everyone the same. No exceptions.

To create and sustain a true human community requires a true leader, not a manager of systems and rules. Human communities are messy. They are organic. There are certainly boundaries and parameters and policies, but in a true human community we struggle every day to find the right answer for this person on this day. We do not consult the rule book, but instead our hearts. We listen to everyone. We get all of the information. We discuss and debate with each other. We cry with each other. We love each other. And then we try to do the right thing, not the easy or expedient thing.

And then we do it again and again. We support each other in our growth, both as individuals and as teams. We learn from our mistakes, and we try to do better.

This kind of community is not available to those stuck in institutional thinking or behavior. It is only available to those who dare to risk. Those great leaders who risk everything to grow themselves and others will be the ones who create a context where a real care community can flourish.

And because you are reading this book, this is your imperative. Let go of your fears and follow the path to mastery, understanding that it is a never-ending journey. You will never attain mastery; you can only approach it. Just as the concert pianist or the landscape artist or the martial artist understands: to elevate the art, you must understand the science. This is your time. You have been called to lead. Let us begin.

CHAPTER 3

Understanding Human Behavior

Three Truths & One Lie

LESSON 9
Truth #1: The Automatic Mind

. . . Now I am throwing off the carelessness of youth
To listen to an inconvenient truth
That I need to move, I need to wake up
I need to change, I need to shake up
I need to speak out, something's got to break up
I've been asleep and I need to wake up now . . .

—Melissa Etheridge, singer/songwriter

What I truly understand about human behavior could be put on the head of a pin. But it fascinates me. I am continually astounded by people and their behavior, sometimes in a positive way and sometimes in a not so positive way. I rarely turn on the television anymore because I choose to avoid hearing some of the not so positive things people are doing to each other. People are making a lot of money with these "reality shows," simply because the "truth" of human behavior is wilder than anyone's imagination. Even my own behavior sometimes astounds me. Every time it does, I am quick to examine it, for I have surrounded myself with truly caring friends and family who will examine it for me, if I fail to do so. But I also examine my own behavior because I have a deep understanding of the power of my position and how what I do and how I behave affects other people. And that impact can either move an organization forward or stop it from growing. If you are in a position of formal or informal authority in a long-term care community (or any organization), you have that power as well.

This, my friends, is an inconvenient truth: If you want to bring about change in your organization or in others, then you first have to change yourself.

And that is a problem, because all human growth is painful. It is hard to look in the mirror and recognize that your own beliefs and behaviors may be causing the problems you are having in your organization or in your own life. As the saying goes, "No pain, no gain!" As I have grown and developed as a human being, self-awareness has served me well. A better understanding of myself has provided me with insights that have helped me grow into a better leader, a better mother and grandmother, a better partner, and a better person for those around me. It has helped me be more successful in my professional life. But I think the way it has helped me the most is in developing a strong definition of self. Through that understanding of myself and my own guiding principles, coupled with my ability to examine my own emotions before deciding how to act, I have achieved a measure of peace that was absent in my younger years. If for no other reason than that, I encourage you to continue your journey of self-discovery. If you choose to be a leader in creating the future of long-term care services, then it is imperative that you examine yourself first.

To embrace self-awareness to be an effective person-centered leader, one must attempt to understand the science of human behavior. What drives behavior, ours and those of others?

As I have attempted to answer that question for myself, I have been led to discover many startling realities about human behavior that I previously did not understand. In fact, I have been guilty in the past of assigning all adult behavior to rational choice, as if we are always in control of our own behavior. This belief has led me to make rash judgments about others' behavior, without truly understanding the impetus or driving factors causing the behavior.

Many of us have played the game "Three Truths and a Lie" at parties, trainings, or conferences. Participants each write down three truthful things and one lie about themselves. The cards are then put in a pile and drawn out one at a time. As each card is read, the group attempts to find the lie among the items listed and then tries to discover who wrote the card. The writer then tells the group if they correctly identified the "lie." It is a great way for a group to get to know each other and can also elicit much laughter as the truths are revealed, each one a little wilder than the next in trying to fool the group.

Because, in fact, most of us know very little about human behavior, I have identified below what I call three "truths" and one "lie" about human behavior that fascinate me as a leader, more than any others:

1. The vast majority of human behavior is directed by things that are happening at a subconscious level, not a conscious level.

2. Human behavior is based more on context than character.

3. Knowledge does not change behavior.

4. As a leader, I need to treat everyone the same.

Unlike the party game, I am not trying to fool you here. The first three are my "truths" and the fourth is the "lie." Take a moment to first ponder the three truths. I say truths because there is an ever-increasing body of research that validates these statements. How do these three truths impact your work as a leader of people?

TRUTH #1: THE AUTOMATIC MIND

Most of us would like to believe that we are in control of our own behavior. We assume that we are rational beings who use our brains to think, analyze, plan, and act. But you will be surprised to know that more often we have very little control over what we do. Our behavior is driven by things happening at a subconscious level, and we are seldom in conscious control.

Even those actions that we believe are a result of conscious thought and decision making can be driven by our emotions, not rational thought. It is generally believed, by many social psychologists, that most of our actions are controlled by the subconscious or automatic mind, and that we are not in control of the actions governed by our subconscious mind. If you Google the word *subconscious*, you will find many images depicting an iceberg. This is intended to illustrate that the conscious mind, like an iceberg, represents the 10% above the water, while the subconscious and unconscious minds represent the 90% below the surface.

This is why I have an internal chuckle every time a formal leader tells me that he needs to be in control. Control is a myth. Not only can we not control the behavior of others, but we are often not even in conscious control of our own behavior. Understanding this can actually help us better understand ourselves and the people around us. It can help us improve relationships with everyone in our lives. It can help us in the all-important journey of self-awareness.

The subconscious controls our central nervous system and many automatic systems that keep us alive. If we had to be aware and make a conscious decision every time we needed to take a breath, we would not be able to do anything else. So our subconscious mind is very helpful. It takes over for us with respect to many tasks that no longer require our full attention. Have you ever driven somewhere and upon arrival realized that you cannot remember getting there? How did you avoid all the potholes and other obstacles? How did you know when to stop and when to go? How did you know how fast to drive or where to turn? Your automatic or subconscious mind got you there safely.

Try this experiment: Take your hand and put it palm up at eye level so you can see what is in your palm. Now picture a lemon sitting in your palm. See it in your mind's eye: a beautiful yellow lemon sitting in your palm.

What do you notice about your mouth? Is it watering?

Your cognitive, rational mind knows there is no actual lemon in your hand. But your subconscious mind, which controls your body's reactions to external events, only knows what you pictured in your mind, as if you actually had a lemon in your hand. Now you have a new trick for your next party.

Your subconscious is more than a party trick. It is actually a powerful force that requires enormous effort to overcome its influence.

THE REALITY MODEL

Watch your thoughts; they become words. Watch your words; they become actions. Watch your actions; they become habits. Watch your habits; they become character. Watch your character; it becomes your destiny. —Lao Tzu

Let us examine the Reality Model (Figure 9.1) as a means of understanding human behavior and the power of our subconscious in determining that behavior. I have adapted this model from

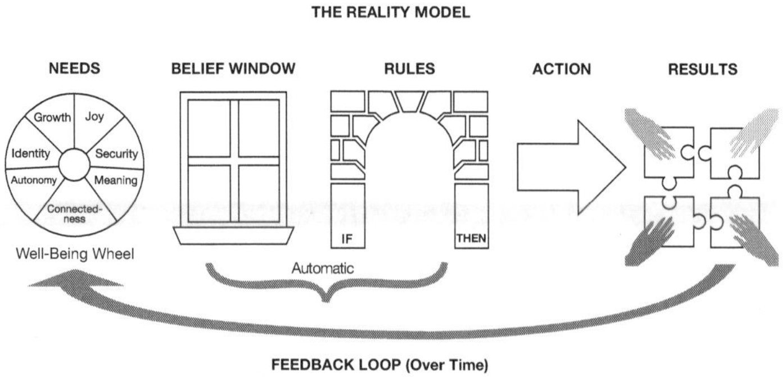

Figure 9.1. The Reality Model. (Adapted with permission from Smith, H. (2013), *The Power of Perception: 6 Steps to Behavior Change.)*

the wonderful work of Hyrum Smith and his book, *The Power of Perception: 6 Steps to Behavior Change.* Smith (2013) has used his version of this model to help many at-risk teens change their own behavior by first changing their beliefs.

We have all heard the saying "perception is reality." Just as you pictured a lemon in your hand and that became a reality through your mind's eye, so it is that many of our perceptions become reality. Through the Reality Model, Smith helps us understand just how true this is, including how our actions are often a result of our perceptions.

Look at the Well-Being Wheel in the Reality Model. These are our needs, and they are shown in the shape of a wheel because they are the drivers. Everything we do is an effort to meet these needs. We all have the same human needs. We come into and leave this world with the same needs, and we are constantly trying to fulfill those needs. I do not care what your title is, where you were born, how old you are, how much education you have had, what gender you are, how much money you make, what your IQ is, or if you drive a Mercedes or ride the bus to work—we all strive for well-being in our lives. For the purpose of understanding the Reality Model, I am using The Eden Alternative Domains of Well-Being™ as the foundational human needs. Figure 9.2 shows them in hierarchy, as adapted by my friend Dr. Al Power in his book, *Dementia Beyond Disease: Enhancing Well-Being* (2014, p. 99). The Reality Model will also work if you use other models for human needs. I delve more deeply into these well-being domains in Lesson 24.

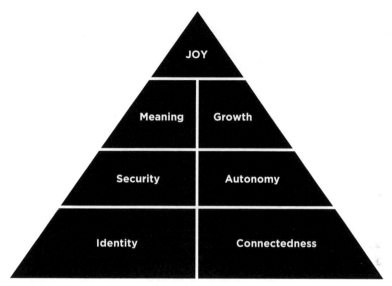

Figure 9.2. The Eden Alternative Domains of Well-being™.

Well-being is the highest outcome of a human life. We all have the same need to experience well-being. As with Maslow's Hierarchy of Needs, as the lower needs are met, we are able to fulfill our higher purpose needs. Once all of our well-being needs are met, we can live in a state of joy. Let us now examine how the Reality Model (Figure 9.1) designs and crafts our behaviors to meet these human needs.

So we all have the same basic needs, but we all come into this world without any beliefs or judgments. Certainly, we are born with a personality that influences our basic tendencies. Anyone who has more than one child or grandchild knows that each child has a personality from the moment of birth. I have two sons whose personalities are completely different, almost total opposites. Those two sons have each given me a grandchild, one a boy and the other a girl. And even though my granddaughter is only 2 years old at this writing, I can tell that my two grandchildren have completely different personalities. (More on personalities later.)

But beliefs are different from personality. Look at the Belief Window in the Reality Model. When we are born, our belief windows are like clear panes of glass. Then, depending on the experiences we have in life, we start to put filters on those belief windows. These filters color the way we see the world. They create our perceptions. Because my grandchildren have different parents, each will have different experiences that will lead to different filters on their belief windows. Because of that, they will each perceive the world differently.

We each have our own life's journey, a journey that we started as a child. We were born into different cultures. We have different parents with different belief systems. We are exposed to different experiences that either support or contradict those beliefs. As a 67-year-old woman born in south Texas and raised by educated, conservative parents, the filters I have on my belief window will most likely be different from those of a 17-year-old boy born in Harlem and raised by a single mother who had to work three jobs to make ends meet.

But both that young boy and I make our own judgments about our own behavior as well as the behavior of others. The problem is that we started making these judgments very early on in our lives when we did not have the capability to truly judge situations. Based on our child-brains, we accumulated some learning and created a knowledge base. We made judgments about ourselves and about the people around us (what type of people are good, what type of people are bad). The longer we live, the more filters get put onto our belief windows, and the more our perceptions become realities. We must recognize that our beliefs can color the way we perceive the world and may not help us in meeting our needs. Unless we bring our beliefs into our conscious mind to fully examine them, we will continue to act based on the filters that create our perceptions.

When we repeat some of our actions, we have subconsciously reinforced our judgments, learnings, and beliefs. If I am a 16-year-old girl who needs connections with my peers to feed my identity need of being "popular" and I believe that if I do not go out and party with them, they will not like me, then I am likely to go out and party. I believe, in the short term, that I am fulfilling a need for connectedness, identity, and joy, when in fact I may be setting myself up for failure.

Now, look at the Rules part of the Reality Model. Just as the experience of driving a car eventually exists in our subconscious mind through frequent repetition, many of the judgments and things we have learned that are a part of our belief window have also become parts of our subconscious mind by repeated re-enforcements before we could analyze them with our mature conscious brain. And then automatically, without any choice, effort, or even realization on our part, the brain creates paradigms or "unconscious rules" about how we see and judge the world based on the filters our experiences put on our belief window (I believe that I am an above-average driver; therefore, I can drive above the speed limit safely). Once a paradigm is created in the subconscious mind, it starts to influence behavior. In other words: *It is from these unconscious paradigms that our actions are driven.*

If I have experiences in my life that lead me to the belief that "hands-on staff are lazy and stupid and need managers to watch over them," then my automatic mind will create a set of rules about hands-on staff that will lead me to not trust staff and to become a controlling, top-down manager. I may have created this belief after hearing my father talk about his employees or I may have had a boss who told me not to trust the staff. Whatever the reason, this belief is now firmly planted in my subconscious and drives my behavior toward hands-on staff. Unless I become aware that my behavior is not meeting my needs and examine the filters on my belief window, then my behavior will continue, even though it is not serving my needs over the long run.

There are two natural laws with the Reality Model that I want you to understand. The first is, *If the results of your behavior do not meet your needs, there is an incorrect belief on your belief window.* The second is, *Results take time to measure.*

Notice the feedback loop in the Reality Model. The results of our action provide us with feedback on whether our needs are being met by that action or not. The Reality Model tells us that those results take time to measure. So that teenage girl may believe that partying with her friends is meeting her identity and connectedness needs in the short run. But in the long run, it is easy to see that she has an incorrect filter on her belief window. In the short run, that micro-manager or fear-based manager may believe his needs are being met by his actions, but over time they will not be. How many of you enjoy being micro-managed? How many of you enjoy being threatened? None of us do. The Reality Model teaches us, *Human growth happens when you are able to examine the filters on your belief window and change them so that new paradigms are created that then lead to new behaviors.*

If you want to change behavior, yours or others', you have to discover the filter on the belief window that is causing that behavior and change that filter. You can certainly use the power of hierarchy to change behavior in the short-term. But if you are looking to change behavior in the long run, you must change the belief that is driving that behavior. *Thus, self-awareness becomes the absolute imperative of an ongoing leadership practice.*

So here is your mirror: What beliefs are driving your own behavior? If the results of your actions as a leader over time are not meeting your needs, then you need to examine the filters on your belief window. Consider if you have any of the following filters:

- There is just no work ethic anymore.

- Hands-on staff is lazy and will only do things right if someone is monitoring them.

- My job is to come up with the answers to solve our problems and tell my staff what to do.

How is that working for you? How do other people perceive you?

And this same process is happening in everyone's brains, not just ours as formal leaders. We must also try to understand the beliefs that may be driving the behavior of our employees. Is that behavior I do not like a conscious choice, or is that behavior being driven by subconscious paradigms formed by false beliefs?

The subconscious mind is a tool that we have not been taught how to use effectively. When we understand its process and how beliefs are driving our behavior, we can begin to examine our beliefs with an adult mind and stop being a victim to our own subconscious.

The next time you are completely frustrated by a staff member's behavior, before you start judging that behavior, take a moment to try to determine what belief might be driving that behavior. Using the Reality Model, we can understand that behavior is driven by things happening on a subconscious level. We can stop blaming and begin examining the ill-founded beliefs that may be influencing the behavior. When we are able to shift the belief, the paradigm changes; when the paradigm changes, our actions change.

That is the lesson of Truth #1.

LESSON 10
Truth #2: Context versus Character

It is practically impossible to understand a thought, an act, a move of any sort from the situation in which it occurs.

—Jerome Bruner, psychologist

Our beliefs are driving our behavior on a subconscious level. That is true. But there are other forces at work in our subconscious minds that shape our behavior as well. One of those is context, which is defined as, "the situation in which something happens; the group of conditions that exist where and when something happens" (Merriam-webster.com).

A multitude of factors can create a context that then influences human behavior. There are cultural, environmental, social, hierarchical, and institutional influences, to mention just a few. There are certainly too many influences in a care community that are affecting the behavior of you and your staff to discuss them all, but I do want to note a few of them:

- Leadership ability and style
- Physical environment
- Organizational structure and design
- Hierarchy
- Conflict and how it is managed (or not managed)
- Institutional thinking and trappings
- Organizational culture and climate
- Fear-based accountability
- Mission, vision, and values
- Relationships

- Surplus safety
- Reciprocity
- Aging as decline
- Scarcity mentality
- Standards of conduct

Throughout this book, I attempt to touch upon many of these from a formal leader's perspective. Because they contribute to context, they also contribute to the behavior of everyone who lives and works within a context. Many of these factors have been driven by our subconscious beliefs. So we will have to bring them into our consciousness to change those beliefs in order to change the context.

In my previous book, *The Journey of a Lifetime: Leadership Pathways to Culture Change in Long-Term Care*, I write about a phenomenon in human psychology called Fundamental Attribution Error (FAE). This is a cognitive bias among many managers in attributing all of the behavior of their staff to the employees' character, rather than the context in which they work. Many managers assume that human character is all-encompassing, and if they can just hire the "right people" (people of good character), then everything would be perfect (Fox, 2007).

I have found this belief is prevalent in long-term care; managers often blame the lack of staff performance on the character of the people they believe they are forced to hire, because "We can't pay enough to hire good people." Look around you. There are amazingly good, courageous, and compassionate people all over long-term care, many working at low wages. If wages were a determination of work ethic and being a "good" employee, where did these people come from? And if making a large salary was a determinant of good character, what happened to Bernie Madoff? Or Kenneth Lay?

In fact, researchers from the University of California, San Diego, and the University of Toronto found that wealthier people are more apt to behave unethically than those who have less money. In these studies, it was found that rich people are more unethical and likely to cheat, break the law, or behave badly toward other people (Piff, Stancato, Côté, Mendoza-Denton, & Keltner, 2012).

The cognitive bias of FAE causes us to not recognize the impact that context has on human behavior. *Context, in fact, influences human behavior far greater than does one's character.* Many social science studies have validated this statement. In his book, *The Tipping Point*, Malcolm Gladwell (2006) shares two stories about helping behavior and how it is greatly influenced negatively by

- the number of people present (in larger groups, helping behavior is diminished)

- whether the person is in a hurry (people in a hurry are much less likely to help)

Put these two factors into the *context* of a large institutional building we have in long-term care and the way staff is always rushing madly about, and it is easy to see why someone walks past a call light or does not clean up a spill on the floor. The institutional model has created a context in which helping behavior is diminished.

Thus, we see efforts by the person-centered care movement to create smallness, even within the larger physical plant, to blend roles through cross-training and the creation of cross-functional teams to improve efficiency and eliminate the need for rushing madly about.

Another famous social science experiment was conducted by Muzafer Sharif in 1954 and also illustrates the power of context on human behavior. Sharif and his associates took a group of 22 11-year-old boys from Oklahoma to a campground in Robbers Cave State Park. The group could not have been any more similar. They were all raised by two parents (mother and father) in rural Oklahoma and held the same values and beliefs.

The bus ride on the way to the camp was uneventful. When they arrived at the campgrounds, the researchers divided the boys into two groups and separated them for a week, after which the boys would be brought back together for a series of competitive games. In only one week's time, the groups both formed their own opposite cultures. One group named themselves the Rattlers while the other group took on the name the Eagles. The Rattlers cursed, and the Eagles prayed and banned cursing. When the groups were brought back together, the trouble started immediately. The Rattlers staked their "flag" on the baseball field and claimed it as "our" field. The Eagles tore it down and burned it. The Rattlers raided the Eagles' cabins, trashed their belongings, and stole some clothing. The Eagles armed themselves with sticks and raided the Rattlers' cabins. They then returned to their own cabins and started putting rocks in their socks preparing for the retaliation they knew would come. These 11-year-old boys, who were all getting along on the bus ride to the campgrounds, became mortal enemies within a week of being separated, to the point they were ready to go to war with the other group (Brooks, 2011).

This experiment showed what dozens of others have confirmed: Human-beings have a tendency to form groups (tribes, constituencies) based on the most arbitrary characteristics imaginable (e.g., night shift, dietary department, staff on B-hall), and when those groups come into contact with each other, there will be trouble.

Can this explain why I can go into any nursing home or assisted living facility that has followed an institutional model of care with the same organizational structure and find the same ongoing, unmitigated conflict happening between the same constituencies? Are these bad people, or have we created a context for conflict through our organizational design, departmental approach to care, and top-down hierarchy?

Understanding this tendency for forming constituencies and how those constituencies will come into conflict, formal leaders are beginning to recognize the imperative for organizational redesign. They understand that we must break out of our constituencies and return to a community. Here is the way I define constituency versus community:

- *Constituency:* a group of people who work to promote their own agenda and fulfill their own needs, often to the detriment of people outside their constituency

- *Community:* a group of unrelated people living and working together in shared fellowship toward a common noble aim

Today we see an enormous effort in long-term care to create cross-functional, empowered teams instead of departments and shifts. In my management organization, Vivage Senior Living, we knew that we would not be able to tear down our old institutional buildings and build Green Houses. We knew we would not be able to even remodel most of our outdated buildings into household models to make this work of organizational redesign easier. So we created a curriculum to help managers evolve. Using 30, 1-hour modules, our Neighborhood Guide curriculum trains managers how to grow cross-functional, self-managed neighborhood teams. We also warned them that through this process, they could easily be trading old constituencies for new ones. As people came out of their old constituencies (departments, shifts, management, staff), they could very quickly form into neighborhood constituencies. We need to recognize that this is our nature as human beings. So it is a Neighborhood Guide's role to help bring all of the teams together into community. If one team fails, they all fail.

We began with five different communities in 2010. Since then, another seven have joined in this effort toward organizational redesign. It is hard work, but all of the communities reported on its value. Our research on the well-being of staff and elders validated those reports. All showed improvement in all of the well-being domains. We also measured empowerment using a tool called the Conditions for Work Effectiveness Questionnaire II (CWEQII). Again, our results were positive and showed an increase in empowerment among all of the pilot communities. The Neighborhood Guide curriculum has been licensed to The Eden Alternative so that other communities wanting to attempt the challenging but rewarding work of changing the context through organizational redesign can use it. I believe it is one pathway to sustainable person-centered care.

Of course, this curriculum requires leaders to change first. Here is another inconvenient truth for leaders in long-term care: You are the *context creators*. You create the context in which all of the behavior of your staff occurs. Some may find that disquieting. I find it hopeful. It is unlikely that I am able to change or even influence anyone's character, but I can change and influence the context of my organization. I can create smallness within the large to improve helping behavior. I can cross-train for efficiency and effectiveness to stop the rushing around, and I can change the organizational design to break down constituencies.

Truth #2 teaches us about the importance of changing the context to change behavior and that formal leaders are the context creators. There are many ways to change the context of an organization by changing leaders' behaviors. I touch on many of these throughout this book. It is important to remember, however, that all change, even contextual change, only becomes sustainable when we change our beliefs (Truth #1). And as you will soon learn about Truth #3, changing behavior takes more than just educating others.

Truth #3: Knowledge Does Not Change Behavior

Knowledge DOES NOT change behavior. You must ACT your way into a new way of thinking.

—Robin Shea, lifestyle transformation coach

One of the responsibilities in my current position is to develop, deliver, and evaluate educational curricula to assist our communities in leadership development and person-centered care. I am an adult-educator. I deal in knowledge. I believe in knowledge. I continue to educate myself so that I can educate others. This work is both exciting and fulfilling to me. Yet, I know that knowledge by itself does not change behavior; if it did, then we would all recycle, exercise, eat right, and save for retirement and no one would ever text and drive. I know that I have written more than a few plans of correction that begin, "We will re-educate . . . "

How many times have you told "them" to do "it" one way, only to have "them" do "it" the way they want to do it? So, we re-educate. And then we re-educate again. And again. And once more. Then we say really stupid things like, "If they would just give us enough money, we could hire the right people!" You have the right people. You just have the wrong context and the wrong filters on their belief windows. So if you want to change behavior and make that behavior change sustainable, you have to change the context and change beliefs. And educate and re-educate, again and again, until the new behaviors become a new habit that replaces the old habit.

In his book, *The Power of Habit*, Charles Duhigg (2012) teaches us that habits influence what we do in life and in business. Habits are the choices that all of us make at some point and then stop thinking about but continue doing, often every day, because the behavior has become automatic. (Remember the automatic mind.)

It is a part of our neurology, the automatic mind, the basal ganglia—the more primitive part of the brain takes over from the thinking part of the brain, the prefrontal cortex. Duhigg helps us see that by understanding how this happens, we can rebuild those habits in whichever way we choose.

The basal ganglia, found at the base of the cerebrum, are the part of the brain that controls automatic behaviors like breathing, swallowing, and the startle response. In the 1990s, researchers at the Massachusetts Institute of Technology (MIT) began studying the basal ganglia and its role in developing habits. To learn more, they studied rats learning a maze. They discovered there is a process by which the brain converts a series of actions into an automatic routine, what they called "chunking." Think about your own routines. We all have them. Our routines have become habits and, therefore, we can manage them without any conscious thought. We are usually thinking about all sorts of things other than what we are doing as we go through our routines.

Research has shown that habits emerge because the brain is constantly looking for ways to save effort. The brain wants to help you out, so it will try to make almost any routine into a habit. This is a great advantage to us as human beings. For one thing, an efficient brain requires less room, which makes for a smaller head, which makes childbirth easier. At least half our population is thankful for that. But the automatic brain has also helped us evolve as a species. It allows us to stop thinking constantly about basic behaviors so we can devote mental energy to inventing tools and technology and to creative pursuits. Michelangelo would never have completed the paintings on the ceiling of the Sistine Chapel if he had not had the advantages of an automatic mind. And you and I would never make it through our morning routines if we had to consciously think about every step.

But we do not want our automatic brains to take over when we might miss something important. The MIT researchers also found that the basal ganglia have devised a system to determine when to let habits take over. It is something that happens whenever a "chunk" of behavior starts or ends. The brain spends a lot of effort at the beginning of a habit looking for a cue that offers a hint of which pattern to use. And at the end of the activity when a reward appears, the brain shakes itself awake and makes sure everything occurred as expected.

Think about your morning routine before you leave for work. The alarm goes off and the "chunk" begins. The brain has its cue. Your automatic brain clicks in and you begin your routine the same way you do it every other morning you go to work. As you go through your routine, your mind is free to explore many other things. You might be thinking about what you need to do that day or where you want go to lunch or even about that new car you want. None of this disrupts your routine. You go through the motions automatically. You finish your routine. Your reward is you are dressed and ready for work. Then just before you walk out the door, you stop and check to make sure you have everything you need. The "chunk" ends and you need to make sure everything went okay. You come out of your automatic mind and examine yourself. Do you have everything you need to take with you? Are your teeth clean? Did you manage to get your earrings on or the same color of socks? Do you have your wallet or purse, your keys? Yep. Everything looks good. Then off you go. You lock the door. Get in the car. And another cue begins another "chunk." You arrive at work and at times cannot even remember how you got there. You made it without anything bad happening even though your automatic mind was in charge. You have your reward. You brain clicks back in. The "chunk" has ended until the next cue emerges.

Duhigg shares with us that researchers have also identified a "habit loop": a three-part process that involves receiving a cue, participating in a routine, and receiving a reward. Over time, this loop becomes more and more automatic. The researchers found that the "cue and reward become so intertwined that a powerful sense of anticipation and craving emerges and a habit is born" (Duhigg, 2012, p. 19). Duhigg pictures the habit loop something like what is shown in Figure 11.1.

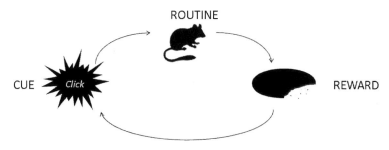

Figure 11.1. The habit loop.

Duhigg reminds us that habits are not destiny; they can be ignored, changed, or replaced. Understanding the habit loop reveals a basic truth: "When a habit emerges, the brain stops fully participating in decision making" (Duhigg, 2012, p. 19). So, unless you deliberately fight a habit and find new routines, the pattern will unfold automatically. This happens every day when you go through your morning routine. And it happens every day when your staff crosses the threshold of your community to work. Walking in that door creates a cue that is so strong their automatic minds kick in. The "chunk" begins and does not stop until they walk out the door.

To change the culture of your community, you have to change the routine, disrupt the context. And you have to do it until a new habit loop is established and that habit becomes automatic.

For decades, formal leaders in nursing homes have been working on the wrong end of the habit loop in an effort to change employee behavior. They have been trying to change the reward, instead of the routine. In my 35 years in long-term care, I have heard of a multitude of different incentives and reward programs. I have tried many of them myself. I am now suggesting that we attack the middle of the habit loop and disrupt the routine. As Duhigg reminds us,

> Habits are powerful, but they are also delicate. They shape our lives far more than we realize. They are so strong that they cause our brains to cling to them at the exclusion of all else, including common sense. They can emerge outside our consciousness, or can be deliberately designed. They often occur without our permission. But can be reshaped by fiddling with their parts. (Duhigg, 2012, p. 25)

Duhigg also alerts us to the Golden Rule of Habits: "You can't extinguish a bad habit, you can only change it" (Duhigg, 2012, p. 63). Use the same cue, provide the same reward, change the routine. By bringing in new habits to replace the old ones, we can change the context of our care communities.

What if we change the context of our care communities to be places where people want to work instead of trying to bribe people into coming to work in places where their well-being needs are not met? I know. It is a radical idea. And it is another inconvenient truth. The truth is that the formal leaders in care communities have to change first. We are the context creators. That means we have to break out of our own habit loops. It means we have to shake off our automatic minds and start behaving differently, building new habits into our daily routines. But what if we could create a context so meaningful and fulfilling that our employees would hear their alarm clock and jump out of bed because the cue and reward of coming to work in our care communities would "become so intertwined that a powerful sense of anticipation and craving emerges and a new habit has been born."

I think that is possible, if we can better understand what motivates us, what our well-being needs are, and how our behavior is driven by beliefs and context, not character. The more we understand about the science of human behavior, the better able we will be in elevating the art of leadership. In Lesson #30, I describe some of the keystone habits that we have used in my company to create new and powerful habits that dramatically changed the context of a care community. These habits have the ability to begin to influence other habits and to create a domino effect that builds a new culture of care. But first, more about human behavior—on to the lie.

The Lie: As a Leader, I Need to Treat Everyone the Same

Treating people the same is not equal treatment if they are not the same.

—Deborah Tannen, linguistics scholar

Employment attorneys preach about the need to treat everyone the same. I wholeheartedly disagree. If I were to do that as a leader, I would be ignoring and denying one of the fundamental truths about human behavior: personality drives our basic behavior tendencies.

It is a fact that we are all the same in many ways. We have the same basic human needs. We have the same human motivators. We share the same emotions. Human beings share 99.9% of our DNA. But that .1% is a doozy.

THE POWER OF PERSONALITY

While some of our personality can be linked to DNA and genetic differences, personality also can be influenced by environmental and experiential factors. Despite how we came to have a personality, we all have at least one. And that personality makes us unique. Personality has a huge impact on how we behave. It makes us who we are. It influences nearly every aspect of our lives, from what we choose to do for a living to how we interact with our families to our choices of friends and romantic partners. It also influences how we communicate.

Knowing this, as a leader, why would I want to treat everyone the same? How is that being person-centered? How is that effectively communicating with an individual? As Deborah Tannen states in the quote above, that's not equal treatment.

Being a person-centered leader means that I understand the power that personality has over how people behave: what stresses them, how they communicate, what their communication needs and mistakes are, and how they will interact with other personality styles. Therefore, it means that I must adjust my behavior to meet the individual needs of each person. Quite a feat! But one worth attempting.

The James Bird Guess International Success Academy is a consulting firm that works with senior leadership teams to improve their effectiveness as formal leaders. In 2015, this group conducted an analysis of "360 leadership feedback data on 1,000 managers, supervisors, and senior level leaders, as well as the most popular leadership training and executive coaching requests and discovered patterns and themes in the 'worst performing' and 'least effective' managers and leaders" (James Bird Guess International Success Academy, 2016).

One of the themes of worst performing managers was that they shared an "inability to adapt to various personality styles." The following is an analysis of this commonality in the worst performing managers:

> They expect and demand employees to adapt to their leadership style. They manage and treat all employees the same way, from high performers to low performers. They perceive others with different communication styles as 'problem players.' When asked too many questions, (especially by new employees) they perceive them as challenging their authority. (James Bird Guess International Success Academy, 2016)

DEEP KNOWING

Being a person-centered leader means that you must know each person so well that you are able to adjust your style to meet his or her needs. This kind of "deep knowing" also runs counter to current human resource practices. "Keep your professional distance," is resounding in my ear right now. Let me say this about relationships in a human community. In every human community, there are personal boundaries that must be maintained. We know what they are in our own communities. Do not cross them. But to be an effective person-centered leader, you must deeply know your staff, and they must deeply know you and each other, as well.

One way that we help facilitate this deep knowing at Vivage Quality Health Partners is by using personality style inventories. It would be nice if we could afford to have everyone take the Myers-Briggs personality inventory, but that has not been realistic for us. So we developed our own personality inventory adapted from many different tools we found for determining personality styles. We think of ours as a sort of "quick and dirty" evaluation. It may not be the most scientifically sound way of determining personality styles, but it works for us. And our employees love to learn more about themselves and their co-workers. This inventory divides us into four different "tree" identities based on a self-test that takes about 30 minutes to complete. Here is a brief breakdown of the four styles:

Oaks: Core value is responsibility. Oaks are traditional, value driven. They have a strong sense of right and wrong. They are task driven and have checklists. They want things done right!

Aspens: Core value is fun. Aspens are people focused. They love to be on stage and on the move. They sometimes over-commit. They can drive an Oak to fits!

Willows: Core value is relationships. Willows are people focused, sentimental, romantic. Willows over-apologize and need a lot of attention. They are great caregivers.

Redwoods: Core value is competence. Redwoods are visionary, logical, and task driven. They are often living in their heads. Although most are caring, they can be perceived as cold and standoffish.

Using this personality inventory with staff in our communities not only helps grow self-awareness of our own personality styles and how we might behave because of those styles, but also helps us understand how we might be perceived based on those styles. It has also helped our teams become deeply known to each other. Knowing someone's personality style gives important cues about how to communicate with the person. This understanding has also, amazingly, helped our staff gain more tolerance of each other. "Oh, right, she's a Willow. That's why she's upset. I need to go apologize."

The following story illustrates how important it is to know these differences in each other:

> I was on the phone speaking to Dr. Bill Thomas about some struggles we were facing in building our new Green House® project in Loveland, Colorado. We were on the phone for over 30 minutes, having a very direct conversation with each other as two Redwoods will do. Less than a minute after I hung up, the phone rang again. It was Bill. He said, "Nance, are we okay?" Confused, I responded, "Yea, Bill. What's up?" He told me that as soon as he got off the phone, his wife, Jude, asked him in a distressed tone, "Who were you talking to?" Bill said, "That was just Nance, why?" Jude said, "Then you need to call her right back and apologize for how you were speaking to her." Bill then said to me, "I thought it might be that Redwood–Willow thing, but I wanted to make sure." Jude is a Willow. When she overheard our conversation, she felt that Bill was speaking rudely to me. Bill and I are both Redwoods. I felt, and so did he, that we were just hashing out some issues together.

That is the power of personality and why we should not buy into the lie of treating everyone the same.

I do want to note one caveat. Personality is an important force in how we behave and communicate. It is not, however, an excuse for bad behavior. As human beings, we have the ability to become self-aware and, using self-discipline, overcome the negative aspects of our own personality. There is no one personality style that is better than the others. All of them have positive and negative aspects. The key is to build upon the positive aspects of your personality style and try to minimize the negative aspects through self-awareness and self-discipline.

I have had employees try to justify their own behavior by saying, "That's just the way I am." And I say, "If you're aware of how you're being a jerk, then change!" I have also worked with a leadership team in a care community that had been using personality styles as a weapon. In this instance, the Oaks were in the majority and were making fun of the Willows for being more emotionally based. Do you see how easily constituencies can form? By facilitating an exercise for this group to discover their personality styles, I had unintentionally created a context for new constituencies. I needed to repair that damage. On my next visit to this community, I explained that using personality style as a weapon is the same as using someone's skin color, nationality, gender, or sexual orientation as a weapon because we do not get to choose our personality. So, as a word of caution, personality styles should never be used as an excuse for your own bad behavior, or as a weapon against others.

Another problem I have with treating everyone the same is that it forfeits the opportunity to transform your community from an institution to a truly caring community. In an institution, everyone is treated the same. "There is no special treatment here!" Those words do not fit in a truly caring community. In a community where each person is well known, there is the opportunity for special treatment for everyone. You may be one of the lucky ones who does not need special treatment, but where would you rather work? In an institution where special treatment is never available or in a community where it is available should you ever need it?

We are all individuals, with unique challenges and talents. To deny that or just ignore it out of our own fear does not make us leaders. Nor does it make us caring. Caring, truly caring, means that I help people to grow. Some people, like some plants, need more nurturing, more time, and more help than others to grow. That is a fact. Treating everyone the same means that those people who may need special treatment will not make it in my community. What a tremendous loss.

I was privileged and challenged to be the project leader for a new Green House development in Loveland, Colorado. Working with the Loveland Housing Authority, we were building six Green House homes on their senior independent living campus. As a start-up, we had to recruit, hire, train, and retain enough staff to operate this new model. This required more than 50 certified nursing assistants (CNAs) who would train to become the *shahbazim* (singular, *shahbaz*; the hands-on care partners in the houses charged with protecting, sustaining, and nurturing the elders). I gained knowledge that one of our new shahbazim was living in a tent with her husband and children. This was August, so the weather was pleasant, but I knew October was just around the corner. I approached the CEO of the housing authority about this issue, and within a week the shahbaz and her family moved into a three-bedroom apartment. I was not afraid that other employees would be mad about this special treatment. It was the right thing to do. Just because none of the other employees needed housing at that time did not stop me from providing special treatment for the one who did. What the other employees did perceive was that if they were ever in need, we would help them. They perceived that we cared about them.

Another story of special treatment also comes from the Green House homes in Loveland. As the six new houses were filled with ten elders each, it became apparent that the care needs in one of the houses exceeded the care needs in the other houses. I asked the new administrator to increase the shahbazim staffing in that house. He was reluctant at first, because he knew that the news would travel fast to all of the other houses. He was concerned of the backlash and having to explain why one house received more staffing. This was a valid concern, but I reminded him that we make decisions based on principles of what is right, rather than succumbing to our own fear. I also suggested to him that if he did get backlash that he could offer that person a position working in the house that needed more staffing. The backlash never came. In fact, he never heard one peep about it. The backlash he expected did not come because everyone on the campus understood the challenges in that house. Ultimately they perceived that we would respond to their needs in the future.

I think it is important for the formal leaders to talk about special treatment. Because there are so many institutional paradigms that color the way people see the world, we need to talk about the reasons for our decision making.

There are many other paradigms formed by the institutional model's belief system that must be broken, to help people see in a different way, if you want to create a person-centered care community. I discuss many of them throughout this book, but I once dealt with an interesting paradigm that I had not encountered before.

In one of the Loveland Green House homes, we had three friends who lived together as well as worked the evening shift together. The shahbazim have to work together across all shifts in this model as a self-managed team. There was some conflict between these three friends who worked the evening shift and the people who worked the day shift; namely, one person working days was not completing her housekeeping tasks. As the shahbazim team talked through issues together, the conflict did not go away. In fact, the person working days tried to make it a shift war by recruiting one other person into her tribe, but she was unable to sway another shahbaz who also worked the day shift.

The women working evenings were growing more and more frustrated, as nothing seemed to change. The guide of the house asked me to meet with the person working days who seemed not to be completing her tasks, as things were getting uglier. (In the Green House model, a guide is a manager to whom the self-managed team of shahbazim report.) In my discussions with this employee, she stated vehemently that people living together should not be allowed to work together in the same house. (There is a belief for you!) I asked her why. She said that because they lived together, they were "ganging up" on the day shift. She stated that she thought we should split the three friends working evenings into different houses. I told her that was an interesting perception, because I had witnessed that she and the other person working days, who did not live together, had managed to "gang up" on the women working evenings. I also stated that I did not believe living together was an issue. If she had a performance issue with her team members, I would be happy to listen to her concerns; their private lives, however, were not up for discussion. She sat silently for a moment. What she and I both knew was that these three friends had no performance issues. In fact, they worked well together because they cared about each other. And their concerns about her were not ill-founded. Ultimately their concerns were for the well-being of the elders they served and for their own success as a team.

I offered her the option of moving to another house if it bothered her that these women lived together. But from what I understood, all they wanted was for her to complete her assignments. And because the entire team worked together to divide the duties in the house, she had a say in how those assignments were divided between shifts. She seemed to be the only one unable to complete her assignments, so if she did go to another house, the expectations would remain the same.

She decided to stay in the house, but had since been invited to leave the community, and the team is doing better. During her time as a team member, I do not think she ever managed to change her belief that people who have relationships outside of work should not be working together. That belief was driving her negative behavior toward her team members. I know, however, that strong relationships like the one the three friends shared are necessary to build a high-functioning team. Human communities have plenty of boundaries to protect us. We really do not need institutional boundaries founded on misperceptions. They only get in our way of creating caring communities.

Human behavior is complex. There are many things that can influence our behavior and that of others. Rarely is behavior a rational choice. If you want to influence others' behavior, you must begin to understand the three truths and one lie. You must understand that human behavior is driven by beliefs, context, habits, and personality. Working to change behavior, and to make behavior change sustainable, *leaders must shift belief, change context, replace routine, and treat people the way they need to be treated to grow as individuals.* Later lessons will translate these truths into real-life practices you can use to create a truly caring community.

Person-centered leaders also need to understand the human brain. We have already explored the subconscious mind and its influence on human behavior. The brain itself is an incredible tool, a complex network that has evolved across millennia. It is not necessary for us lay people to understand the complete workings of the brain; however, some knowledge of the brain and its impact on human behavior can lend credibility to our work of growing ourselves and others. When we begin to understand a little of the workings, we can elevate the art of our own leadership. The lessons in Chapter 4 delve more deeply into understanding how the brain shapes human behavior. So come along and let us explore your brain and the brains of your employees.

Understanding the Human Brain

A Leadership Tool

The Judging Brain & Negative Bias

The human brain has 100 billion neurons, each neuron connected to 10 thousand other neurons. Sitting on your shoulders is the most complicated object in the known universe.

—Michio Kaku, physicist

Since ancient times, the human brain has been a subject of intrigue. Only in the past few decades, with the invention of new technologies and through studies of the brain's activity, are we gaining a better understanding of our own brains.

As a nursing home administrator, I have never taken a class on the workings of the human brain. Sure, I studied psychology, but I really never delved into neurology. I do not imagine that many of us who have chosen the path of long-term care leadership have ever even considered the workings of the human brain in our daily work. And if we have, it has been in relation to the diseases of or trauma to the brain that might bring someone to live in our communities. We have learned about plaques and tangles and how the brain deteriorates as a result of dementia. We have seen some of the behavioral challenges brought on by a traumatic brain injury. Some of us have had residents with major mental illnesses. We have even thought that some of our residents' family members must have something wrong with their brains. But have we ever considered how the brain impacts our behavior and the behavior of our staff?

As noted in Lesson 12, there is a lot going on in our brains on a subconscious level that greatly influences our behavior. And there is a lot more to understand. In this chapter, I touch on a few things I have learned about the brain and its impact on behavior, from the perspective of leading people in the transformation of organizational culture and climate. I have found that the brain is a powerful tool that we can draw upon in our work as formal leaders, but only once we better understand it.

THE JUDGING BRAIN

The first of these understandings is how we continually judge ourselves and others. We have all heard the saying that, "You only get one chance at making a first impression." Why are first impressions so important? What is happening in our brains in those first few moments when we see someone for the first time? And why is that impression more important and lasting in our brains than subsequent interactions with that person? Why do we humans constantly judge ourselves and others? And why and how is that judgment different? These and many other questions about "the judging brain" are being answered through new neuroimaging technology and an increase in research on how our brains impact our behavior.

Previous research, including Todorov, Baron, & Oosterhof (2008), has shown that the brain's amygdala automatically judges a person's trustworthiness when his or her face is clearly visible. From the moment we see someone for the first time, subconsciously we begin to judge that person's trustworthiness. Current research out of the New York University Department of Psychology shows that the amygdala can evaluate that trustworthiness information even without a face being consciously perceived. In an article published in the *Journal of Neuroscience*, a research team led by Jonathon Freeman found that the brain can judge the apparent trustworthiness of a face from a glimpse so fleeting the person has no idea they have seen it (Freeman, Stolier, Ingbretsen, & Hehman, 2014). So, subconsciously, without our awareness, our brains are making these kinds of judgments about a person's level of trustworthiness.

In his book, *Thinking Fast and Slow*, Nobel Prize–winner Daniel Kahneman asserts that when it comes to social perception, our brains use shortcuts, or heuristics, to draw conclusions about another person. There are many shortcuts the mind relies on when it reads facial expressions, body language, and intentions. One of the most powerful shortcuts is called the "primacy effect," and it explains why first impressions are so important. According to the primacy effect, the information that one person learns about another in his early encounters with that person powerfully determines how he will see that person from then on.

Think about that the next time you meet someone for the first time. First impressions, even impressions made without any awareness on your part, can have a lasting impression on how you judge that person. Even judgment outside your awareness is coloring your perceptions of others as well as their perceptions of you.

But even beyond those first impressions, we continue to judge ourselves and others. Everything a person does is then subject to this judgment. The problem is that we judge ourselves and others differently. In his book, *The Speed of Trust: The One Thing that Changes Everything,* Stephen M. R. Covey states "We judge ourselves by our intentions and others by their behavior." This kind of judging breaks trust. As leaders who want to create a caring community, we must become aware of our judging brains and bring into our awareness how that judging might be coloring our perceptions of people. This constant judging creates and perpetuates a lot of the suffering in our communities and in ourselves.

I have begun to change the way I do presentations at conferences. Instead of delivering a PowerPoint presentation and talking at people, I enjoy having participants identify their greatest leadership challenges by writing down a behavior of another person that is driving them crazy. It is surprising to me that most of the time the participants do not write down a behavior. Instead, they write down their judgment of that behavior. I then have to ask questions to reveal the actual behavior that is disturbing to them.

For instance, someone will write, "She doesn't respect my position or authority." That is a judgment of someone else's behavior. I then ask, "What exactly is this person doing that makes you believe she doesn't respect your position or authority?" An answer might be, "She never tells me when she's leaving for her break." The participant has passed judgment on her employee's behavior by forming an assumption. Everything the employee subsequently does is then subject to an interpretation based on that assumption. It happens constantly.

When we can separate the behavior from our own judgment of that behavior, we can begin to clearly see our responsibility in creating our own suffering. When I have asked a participant if she has requested or reminded her employee to tell her before she goes on break, guess what? The answer is usually, "I guess I should do that."

That is just one example of how we judge without even being aware of it. As person-centered leaders, we must stop judging and recognize that we are all good people who are working very hard to create warm, caring, and safe places for our elders. Leaders do that by creating a warm, caring, and safe place for their staff. Go to the place of compassion and curiosity, not judgment.

THE NEGATIVE BIAS

Because of the work that I do and my interactions with many of our employees through trainings, I often find myself faced with their high emotions. When this happens, I challenge them to be responsible for their own feelings. If a consultant or a supervisor reveals to an employee that she may be falling short in an area of her work, the employee often gets emotionally upset and feels as though she is being picked on. In trying to understand why this is, I have come to understand that the human brain has a negative bias.

Our brains are tools that help us to anticipate and overcome dangers, protect us from pain, and solve problems. So dangers, pain, and problems are what capture the brain's attention. In his book, *Buddha's Brain*, neuropsychologist Rick Hanson refers to this response as "the brain's negativity bias." The human nervous system, he writes,

> scans for, reacts to, stores, and recalls negative information about oneself and one's world. The brain is like Velcro for negative experiences and Teflon for positive ones. The natural result is a growing—and unfair—residue of emotional pain, pessimism, and numbing inhibition in implicit memory. (Hanson, 2009, p. 41)

Understanding this negative bias when faced with an employee's high emotions, I will often ask the employee if her consultant or supervisor had anything positive to say. The response is often delayed as she tries to re-create the event in her mind, but usually the response is "Yes, my consultant said this . . . was going well." I then ask if she thinks the consultant or supervisor is a bad person. This is usually met with a definitive "No!" I then ask if she believes that the consultant or supervisor was intentionally trying to hurt her feelings, and usually the response is also no. I will then ask the employee if she had hurt someone else's feelings, what would she want that person to do. I am always told, "I would want them to tell me so I could apologize." To which I respond, "Then I hope you would give your consultant or supervisor the benefit of the doubt and tell her how you feel. She'll probably want to apologize. Then you can tell her how best to deliver negative information to you in the future, so that it won't hurt your feelings."

Coaching people to manage their own emotions is a large part of my job. We are blessed to work with very caring, emotionally based people. They have big hearts, and those big hearts are easily broken. Combine that with the negative bias of the brain and a fear-based institutional system and you have the formula for a lot of unnecessary suffering. It does not matter whether you work in a caring community or a corporate office, these feelings will get in the way of seeing clearly unless we are able to take responsibility for them.

Because our brains have a negative bias, as leaders we must be very careful about how we deliver information that may be perceived as negative. I have given performance reviews to individuals who were wonderful employees. I laud them at every turn. But when I mention one growth opportunity to someone, that is all the person remembers about the entire review. The opportunity for growth is perceived instead to be a failure.

It is the job of a manager to help people to grow. We must point out those opportunities. But how we do that can make or break someone's spirit. Most people know their own shortcomings, so I have now begun asking people to complete a self-assessment that I review and then discuss with them. I also try to leave them with the positives, instead of giving all of the positives first and leaving the growth opportunities for last. In one training, a director of nursing told me that she uses the "Oreo" method when evaluating staff: she sandwiches the growth opportunities between praise.

But considering our brain's negative bias, I need be mindful of more than just changing the way I share growth opportunities. I also need to be aware of everything I say, the tone of my voice, and my body language in every interaction I have with staff. I know people are watching me and looking for my approval. Because of my position, I have the ability to make or break their day. I also talk about negative bias with staff and challenge them in their own thinking. Then I invite them to help me if I fall into negative bias.

LESSON 14
Emotional Contagion

If we think about emotion this way—as outside-in, not inside out—it is possible to understand how some people can have an enormous amount of influence over others. Some of us, after all, are very good at expressing emotions and feelings, which means that we are far more emotionally contagious than the rest of us.

—Malcolm Gladwell, journalist

Every nursing home in the United States has an infection control program that attempts to mitigate the spread of any type of infection that may arise. We understand the dangers of living and working within close proximity to many others, and we understand the frailty of many of our residents and their susceptibility to infection. We have process improvement committees that track and trend infections and conduct root-cause analysis and action planning to reduce the risk of infection in the human body.

But have we considered that our employees and residents are also susceptible to emotional contagions? Emotional contagion is the idea that emotions are contagious, just as bacteria and viruses are contagious. We can actually "catch" happiness, anger, fear, or virtually any emotion from other people. We have all seen it happen in our care communities. A group may be in a wonderful mood, but then one person in a foul mood joins in, and the mood of the entire group changes almost instantly. We most certainly have seen the impact of emotional contagion on our employees when the state surveyors arrive. A virtual pall consumes the community, driving stress levels through the roof.

As I am writing this in 2016, I am reminded of this phenomenon of emotional contagion as it applies to an entire country. Great Britain's populace voted to exit the European Union, an astounding event that took the leadership of the United Kingdom by surprise. They completely underestimated the emotional contagion that had invaded the country and had driven people to this historic vote. While also threatening the world economy, the event had in one day severely damaged Britain's economic viability, driving the British pound to its lowest level in 35 years.

While much research has been conducted on emotional contagion between two people, research by Sigal Barsade (2002) has shown the significant impact it has on groups as well. Using business school students as subjects for his study, Barsade had them conduct a role-play as department managers advocating for a merit-based pay raise for an employee. All of the students were also part of a "salary committee" given limited resources to allocate. As a part of a committee, they had to negotiate salary increases for everyone, including for their own employee. They each needed to balance the raise for their own employee with the pay raise decisions for all employees to the maximum benefit of the company. Barsade had 29 of these different groups acting as managers on a salary committee. Unbeknownst to the students, Barsade placed "confederates" onto each of the salary committees. These confederates were actors whose job it was to introduce one of four different moods into the groups: cheerful enthusiasm, serene warmth, hostile irritability, and depressed sluggishness.

The findings of his study reveal the enormous impact of emotional contagions. The groups in which a positive emotion was introduced not only had an increase in positive mood, but also showed "more cooperation, and less interpersonal conflict, and felt they performed better than the other groups." Strikingly, these groups actually made decisions that shared the money more equitably. These groups had no idea that their mood had been manipulated by the actor. When queried as to why they thought the group performed the way it did, they gave credit to their own negotiating skills or the qualities of the employees they had been assigned (Barsade, 2002).

As person-centered leaders, we must become aware of the emotional contagions that are infecting our care communities. Unfortunately, in many care communities there seems to be more negative than positive energy, and research shows that negative emotions are more likely to infect others than positive ones (Cacioppo, Gardner, & Berntson, 1997). This, again, is negative bias. Negative emotions are stickier and more contagious. Psychological and organizational research has shown that negative events evoke stronger and quicker emotional, behavioral, and cognitive responses than neutral or positive events (Taylor, 1991).

Armed with this knowledge of emotional contagions and their impact on our performance as a team, we leaders can begin to introduce more positive mood contagions into our communities. We can also mitigate the negative mood contagions through changes in our practices and expectations. I speak to many of these in subsequent lessons.

I have spent the past 20 years working in team development, with teams within my own organization and as an outside facilitator of team process. This experience has given me the ability to read the "mood" of a team very quickly. I do not know how I do this, and I could not teach someone else how to if I had to. It reminds me of what it takes to become a chicken-sexer, a skill that is not easily taught. You and I could look at a baby chick and have no idea of its gender. It takes years of study to master this skill. And master chicken-sexers cannot teach novices how to do it. That is why chicken-sexing is a highly paid job.

So it is with this skill I have developed. Reading the mood of a team, a person, or a community has only come from experience. I have also learned that a team cannot proceed with any degree of effectiveness if its mood is not positive.

I was conducting coaching training with a leadership team in one of our communities. As we were engaging in a pretty intense curriculum, the administrator left the room to attend to a matter. I felt the mood shift almost immediately. Coincidentally, we were discussing the dysfunctions of a team at that time. I allowed my co-trainer to continue the discussion, and I walked out of the room. I was out of the room for a couple of minutes. When I returned, the administrator was still absent. Those present had told my co-trainer that they had a high-trust team and that they could easily address conflict and express disagreement among the team members. I asked the team if they ever disagreed with the administrator. I received a lot of yes nods. I then asked the team if they were able to openly and freely express that disagreement with the administrator. No one would look me in the eye. I now understood the mood shift when the administrator walked out.

This was a team that loved and respected their administrator. They "cared" for him so much that they would not disagree with him or tell him if he was falling short. They wanted to be a high-functioning team, but they did not want to "rock the administrator's boat." I challenged them to open up to their administrator. I knew him and knew he would want to know their feelings. I knew he would want to grow. I also knew that this team was not going to learn anything else that day until this issue could be brought out into the open and resolved. My co-trainer and I left so that when the administrator returned, they could have that discussion. I heard later that it went well.

I tell you that story so that you can begin to see the importance of becoming aware of group mood. I wish I could teach you how to do it, but it is really a matter of "tuning in" to mood and emotions and recognizing the impact they have on our performance as individuals and teams. And it is a whole lot easier than sexing chickens.

We are social beings. Our emotions often drive our behavior. And our emotions are susceptible to others. As a person-centered leader, you must become self-aware of your own mood, tone of voice, body language, and words. If your mood is negative, leave the building until you can get an attitude adjustment. Come back with a positive mood, and infuse that positivity into your community. Become emotionally contagious in a good way. This will require some self-discipline on your part. So let us learn more about that.

LESSON 15
Self-Discipline: The Elephant & the Rider

Self-discipline is not restriction: it's a path to freedom.

—Joseph Rain, spiritual thinker

In his book, *The Happiness Hypothesis,* Jonathon Haidt helps us to better understand our own psychology by explaining how the mind is divided into parts that sometimes conflict with each other. He discusses four different divisions of the mind: mind versus body, right versus left, old versus new, and controlled versus automatic. For our purposes, I focus on controlled versus automatic.

Throughout this book, I have written about the automatic subconscious brain and its enormous impact on our thoughts, beliefs, judgments, and behaviors. Hundreds of subconscious, automatic processes are happening in our brains all the time. The controlled, conscious mind, however, can only handle one process at a time.

We like to believe that we can multitask, but if more than one of those tasks requires our conscious mind, we cannot do it. You cannot listen to someone and work on your computer at the same time. If someone needs to speak with you, you stop what you are doing and give that person your full attention or you will miss something and suffer the consequences later, as I have many times in my life.

Haidt uses a metaphor to help describe these two types of processes. He describes automatic processes as a large elephant and controlled processes as a small rider on the back of the elephant. The rider represents our conscious, thinking, rational brain. Haidt describes this conscious controlled thought as an advisor and servant to the elephant. The elephant "includes the gut feelings, visceral reactions, emotions, and intuitions that comprise much of the automatic system" (Haidt, 2006, p. 17). To put it simply, the elephant is our emotional being, which is housed in the limbic system of the brain. The rider is our rational thinking brain, which is housed in the prefrontal cortex of the brain, the seat of reason. This is where our executive control or self-discipline lives. Haidt explains that the elephant and the rider do not always work well together.

As human beings, we do have some measure of control over our emotions. Our riders can and do make rational choices driven by reason rather than emotion. But different people have different abilities or strengths when it comes to self-discipline. Some people are able to hold the reins of the elephant tighter than others. But in the long run, in any battle between the rider and the elephant, the elephant always wins. As Haidt reminds us: "It's hard for the controlled system to beat the automatic system by willpower alone; like a tired muscle, the former soon wears down and caves in, but the latter runs automatically, effortlessly, and endlessly" (Haidt, 2006, p. 18).

There have been dozens of studies on willpower or self-discipline. Many researchers now believe that our ability to self-manage our rider is like a muscle. And because it is like a muscle, it gets tired. All of us spend time during the day exercising that rider muscle. We bite our tongues instead of speaking our minds. We order a salad instead of a burger and fries for lunch. We suppress our urge to choke an employee who calls off work for the fifth time in 2 weeks. We force a concerned look when a crazy daughter comes in the office to tell us we are killing her mother. All day long, that muscle is getting exercised.

Research shows that interacting with others and maintaining relationships actually depletes our rider muscle (Vohs, Glass, Maddox, & Markman, 2011). You and your employees are highly susceptible to this kind of depletion, which may be why we go home after a stressful day and yell at our kids and eat a pint of ice cream. Our rider muscle is depleted. Our willpower is exhausted.

In his book, *The Power of Habit: Why We do What We Do in Life and Business*, Charles Duhigg shares dozens of studies of how willpower has been shown to be the single most important determinant of individual success, even greater than intellectual talent (Duhigg, 2012). Think about why you are successful in this modern world. How have you made it to your professional position? How have you been able to maintain valuable relationships that make your life better? How have you managed to not choke someone in a fit of rage or not cuss out your boss? How have you been able to come to work even when you are tired, stressed, or having personal problems? It is because you have developed your rider muscle. You have the ability to pull back from your emotions and decide how you want to behave before you act.

How did you grow your rider muscle? Were you fortunate enough to have parents or grandparents who modeled self-discipline and held you accountable for your actions? Did you have teachers who believed in you and helped you deal effectively with your emotions? Have you had mentors, friends, or bosses who helped you with self-control?

Research on willpower and self-discipline has shown us that because willpower is like a muscle, it can be developed. You can strengthen your rider muscle by using it until it becomes a habit. And we know from the research on habits that once a habit is formed, the conscious mind stops fully participating in the activity and it, therefore, becomes automatic and easier. It looks effortless. Somewhere along your life's path, you have benefitted from people who helped you grow into the habit of self-discipline.

I am guessing, however, that not every employee in your care community has had that benefit. I am also guessing that many of the people you are honored to work with are highly emotional people. They feel things more deeply than others. That is what makes them good caregivers. They have big hearts. But because they have big hearts, they also have high emotions. Couple that with weak rider muscles, and you have a situation where the elephant often runs amok.

Recognizing the potential for high turnover due to a lack of self-discipline, Duhigg identifies a handful of companies who are succeeding in helping their employees strengthen their rider muscles. Starbucks is one of these companies. Starbucks relies on entry-level workers who must provide excellent customer service in extremely busy and rushed environments. Starbucks has to convince people to spend $5.00 on a cup of coffee. They cannot have workers who lose it because a customer is rude to them. They rely on workers who can work long hours on their feet and deal with stressful situations. They rely on workers who may not have had the benefit of good role models to help them grow their rider muscles. Does this sound familiar?

How does Starbucks teach their workers to become reliable managers? They listened to the research that shows that self-discipline is not a skill. It is more like a muscle. Because it is like a muscle, if you strengthen self-discipline in one part of your life, that strength will filter over into all parts of your life. Starbucks has spent millions of dollars developing self-discipline in their employees. In the first year of employment, Starbucks' employees spend "at least 50 hours in Starbuck's classrooms, and dozens more at home with Starbuck's workbooks and talking to the Starbuck's mentors assigned to them. The solution, Starbucks discovered, was turning self-discipline into an organizational habit" (Duhigg, 2012, p. 130).

Employees with willpower lapses have no trouble doing their jobs most of the time. The trouble occurs when their rider muscles get depleted when they are faced with unexpected stresses or uncertainties. These employees need a routine to follow when the elephant is taking control and about to charge. So Starbucks created manuals that teach them how to respond to specific cues that might introduce stress into their work day. Stress cues might include a long line of customers, a customer who yells at them, or the temptation to go out and party the night before work. Then managers role-play with employees, teaching a different response to a specific stress cue, and they continue role-playing until the self-disciplined response becomes automatic (Duhigg, 2012).

Willpower can become a habit when employees choose a certain response behavior ahead of time and follow that routine when the actual stressor occurs. What are some of the stress points that often trigger a lapse in self-discipline among your employees? Help them identify those triggers, and create a new routine for them to follow the next time they are faced with that trigger. Role-play the new response with them until it becomes an automatic habit. Provide them with mentors who can coach them as they develop their rider muscles. You can also engage the elders in your community in this effort of helping staff grow their rider muscles. Assign new employees an elder mentor and peer mentor who will help them in forming these new habits. Investing your time in this effort up front will save you time in dealing with the consequences of the elephant stampede we often encounter in our care communities.

LESSON 16
Abundance versus Scarcity

Abundance is not something we acquire. It is something we tune into.

—Wayne Dyer, philosopher

How much of your care community has every available space crammed full of junk? I am guessing that you have so much stuff you do not even know what you have. How many of you have storage sheds in the back of the community filled to the brim with old equipment, mattresses, broken walkers and wheelchairs, leg rests, broken carts, and outdated supplies? Do you know why no one ever throws anything away? Do you know why CNAs hoard linens and supplies? I do. You are living with a scarcity mentality. That scarcity mentality has been perpetuated and passed down for decades from bosses who shared the same mentality.

THE SCARCITY MENTALITY

A scarcity mentality is a belief that one does not have enough . . . of anything. I do not have enough money, resources, time, food—you fill in the blank.

The sad news is that scarcity thinking runs rampant throughout our care communities. And because of our negative biases and emotional contagion, when one person falls into scarcity thinking, others do as well. It is contagious. "So what?" you might ask.

I recommend all leaders read *Scarcity: The New Science of Having Less and How It Defines Our Lives*. Based on the cutting-edge research of Sendhil Mullainathan and Eldar Shafir, this provocative book reveals how scarcity creates a distinct psychology for everyone struggling to manage with less than they need. According to Mullainathan and Shafir, busy people fail to manage their time efficiently for the same reasons the poor and those maxed out on credit cards fail to manage their money. The dynamics of scarcity reveal why dieters find it hard to resist temptation and why students and busy executives mismanage their time. Their research also reveals that regardless of what you believe you are in scarcity of, that belief, that mindset actually impacts your brain. Scarcity imposes itself on the mind at a subconscious level.

In their multiple research studies on this topic, Mullainathan and Shafir examined something they call "bandwidth," which they describe as "Fluid Intelligence, a key resource that affects how we process information, plus Executive Control, a key resource that affects how impulsively we behave" (Mullainathan & Shafir, 2013, p. 13). According to the authors, bandwidth equals the combination of available IQ + self-discipline (that Rider muscle). Interestingly, they found that people who have a scarcity mentality experience a "bandwidth tax." So scarcity mentality generates an internal disruption that directly reduces bandwidth. This is not a person's inherent capacity, but rather how much of that capacity is currently available for use. Scarcity thinking, therefore, not only reduces our cognitive capacity by as much as 14 IQ points, but also reduces our executive control, or our self-discipline (the Rider).

I want to remind you about the power of context on human behavior. If the formal leaders in a care community have a scarcity mentality, it creates a context of scarcity throughout the community that puts a bandwidth tax on every person who lives, works, and visits there.

Another startling result of the study is that scarcity thinking actually creates scarcity, which then drives behaviors we do not like, such as hoarding. Understanding this, leaders in long-term care need to be very diligent in not falling into a scarcity mindset or letting others fall into one.

I believe some of the most dangerous things a formal leader can say are "We can't afford . . . "; I don't have time for . . . "; or "We don't have enough . . . ." These kinds of statements create a perception of scarcity that can lead staff to believe that you do not care. Instead of falling into that scarcity belief, help people believe that the answers to all of our problems are waiting right here in the care community to be discovered. If someone wants to buy something not in the budget, sit down with her and ask, "If you believe this is important, then how can we make this happen? Where can we reduce in other areas to make this a reality?" And, please, stop locking up the supplies! That sends not only a message of scarcity, but also the absolutely wrong message of "I don't trust you."

I worked once with a wonderful community in Oklahoma. As I was conducting a climate assessment, I learned that in order to get supplies after hours or on the weekends, the nursing staff had to call the night watchman, who was the only person on campus with a key to the nursing supplies. This person happened to have a less-than-delightful demeanor, so interacting with her was not pleasant. This created a lot of problems, including frustrated staff, who could not get the supplies they needed to care for their elders, and loss of precious time. It also created the perception that management did not care. I knew the leadership of this community, and this was not something they would have wanted. They were generous, caring people who wanted only the best for their elders. They were not aware of this condition in their community. Once I told them about it, it was remedied immediately. But a scarcity mentality had been created by a broken system that leadership was unaware of. How had that scarcity mentality affected other areas of the community? And was it remedied by correcting the access to supplies? I doubt it.

I recognize scarcity mentality all the time in people who work in our care communities. Usually it is expressed in terms of time and a feeling of being overwhelmed. I now understand how that perception can have a devastating impact on their "bandwidth." The perception of not having enough time not only diminishes intellectual capacity, but also taxes the self-discipline muscle. To mitigate this, one of the exercises I do with both managers and hands-on staff is to ask them to write down their "time stealers." What is taking them away from what is most important? What frustrates them and steals their time? As a team, we go through the time stealers one by one and discuss how to remedy them.

Some of the time stealers mentioned always amaze me, and some of the solutions are so simple that we can eliminate the frustration almost immediately. Someone has been suffering silently, sometimes for years, about something so simple to alleviate it is astounding. Others, of course, take more time to remedy, but we come up with a plan for the team, which brings hope instead of despair. It is rare that the team, working together and with help from the administrator or managers, finds something that cannot be mitigated.

There are only two ways I know how to "make time." One is to build high-trust teams that function extremely well together. Everything is easier in a high-trust environment, and it is crucial to helping people out of their scarcity thinking about time. (I write more about the importance of trust in Lesson 26.) The other is to cross-train. The institutional model uses a division of labor that is inefficient. Cross-training builds capacity and eliminates waste. I am talking about cross-training of everyone, not just hands-on staff. When you have high trust and a multi-skilled team, you can eliminate a lot of the frustration and scarcity mentality that plague our care communities.

THE ABUNDANCE MENTALITY

Person-centered leaders adopt an abundance mentality and foster that mentality in their staff. They are observant of any expressions of scarcity thinking and are quick to squelch it. They hold learning circles to ask staff what is stealing their time (see Lesson 30). They refrain from words that promote a scarcity mentality, and they learn to ask questions that will help them discover the context within their communities that is creating a perception of scarcity.

Abundance thinking opens up possibilities and induces creativity. It primes people to think positively, creating a sense of well-being and hope. Person-centered leaders believe that the answers to all of their problems are right there in their communities waiting to be discovered. They refuse to fall into scarcity thinking and encourage their staff to find solutions together, instead of waiting for a manager to direct them. Abundance thinking is the pathway of growth and opportunity that creates a context for success.

LESSON 17
Hope versus Fear

Hope is the pillar that holds up the world.

—Pliny, the Elder

Fear has been and continues to be used as a means of motivating human behavior. Politicians in the United States on both sides of the aisle use fear to motivate us to vote for them instead of their opponents. Republicans use fear of big government and taxation as a motivator, while Democrats use fear of big corporations and the income gap to scare people into voting their party lines.

Tyrants and oppressive regimes have used fear throughout human history to try to control people. Adolph Hitler engendered fear through the Nazi regime to persecute and murder 6 million Jews in an attempt to transform German society into one master Aryan race. Even religious leaders have attempted to use fear to motivate people as a means of changing behavior.

Marketers use fear as a motivator as often as they can. They present a scenario they hope will invoke our sense of fear. Then they show us a solution, a path back to our comfort zone, that entails using their product or service. All types of media use fear as a means of gaining market share. Parents even try to use fear as a means of controlling their children's behavior.

One might say that in our daily lives fear is in abundance. More importantly for the purposes of our work, we need to understand that *fear is no stranger to long-term care.* Formal leaders also frequently use fear in an attempt to control staff behavior. Just the phrase, "The state is here," causes professional men and women to forget everything they know about their work and make mistakes they normally would not make. For decades, formal leaders in long-term care have tried to use fear of regulators as a means to motivate staff to do things the way they want them to be done.

Many also use the fear of termination and "write-ups" on an almost daily basis. Fear has become a way to manage staff.

THE PROBLEM WITH FEAR

Motivation by fear produces very short-term results, and when faced with fear, employees will leave as quickly as they can. Fear does motivate, but not in a positive way. Fear crushes the human spirit and strips us of our ability to take risks, be creative, adapt to change, and engage in anything more than just the basics of trying to stay out of trouble. Motivation through fear will not produce sustainable results.

Fear is overrated as a motivator because it is disrespectful and demoralizing. Think about the last time fear motivated you to do something well, to exceed your limits, or to really contribute. I am guessing you will not recall a positive experience. Fear does not inspire loyalty, creativity, or genuine commitment. It is a waste of time. No, even more than that. It creates a climate that will lead to your own failure.

And do not think for one minute that the fear you are putting onto your staff is not bleeding over onto your elders. Security, feeling safe and living without fear, is a basic human need. Without it, we cannot achieve any degree of well-being.

As a formal leader, falling into your own fear is just as harmful to your organization as dealing in fear-based tactics. Yes, there is a lot to fear in our world. But as Franklin D. Roosevelt said, "The only thing we have to fear is fear itself." When formal leaders fall into fear, it creates a context in which their behavior becomes more controlling and fear based. When they allow their own insecurities and external threats to dominate the landscape of their community, they create a climate in which growth and change are impossible.

When I mentor administrators, I often tell them that they need to be the "shit dams." Not a politically correct identity, but one that conjures up a powerful image of what I am trying to convey. There will always be outside influences on our care communities, and they often come as negative, fear-inducing threats. One of the most important duties of a person-centered leader is to stop what rolls onto them from rolling down onto their staff or residents. They need to be the "shit dams."

REFRAMING THE FEAR

Besides changing their own behavior, there are three main fear-inducing factors that must be addressed by formal leaders if they hope to stem the tide of fear in their communities:

1. The state

2. The corporate consultants

3. The families

None of these groups are the enemy—the enemy is the institutional model. For decades, formal leaders have made the state the enemy, because the surveyors control what the profession has defined as our greatest measure of success: a deficiency-free survey. I have personally been in many "zero-deficiency" facilities where I would not want to live. This can no longer be our greatest measure of success. Why would we want to live and die on such an arbitrary sword anyway? Our greatest measure of success in the new person-centered culture of care is the well-being of the people who live and work in and visit our communities.

Formal leaders must change the context by teaching staff that the state surveyors are part of our quality improvement team, not the enemy or anything to fear. State surveyors simply bring new eyes into our community to help us see where we can improve. While they are with us, we help them get the information they need to do their jobs as quickly as possible. We do this because we understand how disruptive the process can be to our elders and their care partners. When they leave, we thank them. Then we go to work correcting the things that they found to help us improve.

In Lesson 18, I discuss how the most successful leaders embrace and honor the work of their corporate consultants. These leaders help everyone in the organization see that the consultants are part of the team by embracing and appreciating what consultants bring to the care community, rather than creating a great divide between corporate and facility staff. Great leaders lessen the fear while creating a dynamic context in which each person can grow to his or her greatest potential. Consultants can be a big part of that growth.

Person-centered leaders also embrace their residents' families as partners in providing care; they are not enemies. The "good" families are the ones who are there often challenging us to be the best we can be, not the ones who never complain. A good family member complains to you. That is a gift. With that complaint, the family member is saying, "I trust you to fix this." When we embrace that belief, we can become care partners with them, rather than combatants.

Formal leaders must understand the destructive force that fear has in their organizations and do everything in their power to remove it if they hope to achieve any semblance of a caring community. This is changing the context. Real leaders do not engage in fear. *They deal in HOPE.* There is powerful research on the effects of hope. For decades we have known the healing effects of hope, but more and more research suggests that hope might be the most important feeling we can experience. Studies reveal that hope is the key to good health, the predictor of a meaningful existence, and an indicator of successful performance.

Cutting-edge psychological research, spearheaded by Anthony Scioli, Ph.D., a professor of psychology at Keene State College in New Hampshire, shows that hope is a skill you can acquire. It is active—you can cultivate and nourish it. It is multifaceted—there are 14 distinct aspects, according to Scioli. It is self-perpetuating—hopeful people tend to be more resilient, more trusting, more open, and more motivated than those who are less hopeful. They are likely, therefore, to receive more from the world, which in turn makes them more hopeful—which is why hope is so important. (Scioli & Biller, 2010).

———

In Lesson 7, I shared the story of how I learned about the power of hope from an amazing leader, Sister Amadeus. She had every opportunity to fall into fear and doubt, but somehow rose above it all to create a context of love and hope in the care community she ran. Creating a context of hope instead of fear can dramatically change the culture and habits of your organization. Replacing the fear-based system that exists in most nursing homes may be the person-centered leader's most important job. For when we have a climate and culture steeped in hope, all things become possible and people can explore greater possibilities. *Hope is the pillar that holds up the world.*

CHAPTER 5

Understanding the Problem

*Creating Sustainable
Person-Centered Care*

LESSON 18
Emergent Systems

I really don't know clouds at all.

—Joni Mitchell, singer/songwriter

If we are going to truly transform our institutions into caring communities, then we need to better understand the problem of how to create sustainable person-centered care. As formal leaders in a rapidly evolving system, understanding the science of leadership will not help you if you do not fully understand the problem you are attempting to address through that leadership.

I have been a part of the "culture change movement" for a while. I was one of the early adopters. Show me a cliff, and I will jump off it and grow wings on the way down. That is the courage we needed 20 years ago when the status quo thought we were crazy hippies with this wild idea of changing the culture of care communities.

Many good people have joined the movement and have tried to find the "magic pill," or as I call it "the shiny object," that will instantly change the culture of their communities. There have been many brave people who have attempted to create person-centered care through a programmatic approach. There is the dining program, the bathing program, the horticultural program, the end of life program, and so on. There is restraint reduction, removing alarms, liberalizing diets, and consistent staff assignments. We also have the Artifacts of Culture Change, which was developed by my friends Karen Schoeneman and Carmen Bowman. All of these efforts are worthwhile and have improved the lives of elders living in care communities. Currently, the new shiny objects are music and memory and the virtual dementia tour. I have no problem with any of these efforts. They are important and useful parts of our movement.

My issue is that unless we, the leaders of our care communities, truly understand and address the problem of how to create caring communities, we will never approach a truly sustainable transformation. There is no "shiny object" or "magic pill." Programs are great, but they will go away when the person driving them goes away. The Artifacts of Culture Change have given people the steps to take on this work, but will they lead to the true transformation of our institutions into places where you or I can live and thrive? Will they remove the fear a mother has when she says to her daughter, "Whatever you do, don't put me in a nursing home?" Personally, I do not think so. Only a deep understanding of the problem of how to create caring communities will get us there. And then it will require a willingness on the part of the people who have made this work their careers to change themselves.

Let us begin to understand the problem by looking at organizational change as an emergent system. Consider the difference between clocks and clouds. The philosopher Karl Popper observed there are cloud problems and there are clock problems. A clock is something that is easy to understand. Clocks are "neat, orderly systems that can be solved through reduction." You can take a clock apart and examine its parts to see how it works. If it is not working, you can easily determine the problem and repair the broken part or replace it. Programmatic approaches to transforming the culture of our care communities have been addressing the problem of organizational culture as if it were a clock.

A cloud, on the other hand, is not so easily understood. Clouds are "highly irregular, disorderly, and more or less unpredictable." You cannot take a cloud apart. You have to examine it as a whole. If a cloud is not working, you cannot just fix the parts. A cloud is an emergent system. It has emerged out of a confluence of multiple interactions and there are no direct causal links to follow. A cloud has a dynamic complexity that is not easily understood. You cannot change a cloud. You have to replace it with a new cloud.

In his book, *The Social Animal,* David Brooks helps us to understand what emergent systems are: "Emergent systems don't rely upon a central controller. Instead, once a pattern of interaction is established, it has a downward influence on the behavior of its components" (Brooks, 2011, p. 109). Brooks uses the example of an ant colony as an emergent system. He discusses a study by Deborah Gordon of Stanford University, who discovered that ants all build their colonies the same way. Along with the colony, ants also build a cemetery and a garbage dump, both of which are as far away as possible from each other and the colony, depending on the environment. There is no one "engineer ant" who figures out the geometry and draws a blueprint for the other ants to follow. There is no way each individual ant can even conceive of the entire structure. But individual ants follow "local cues," and other ants adjust to those cues. It does not take long for a precedent to be determined, and once determined, that precedent can last for generations.

Brooks tells us that emergent systems are all around us. The brain itself is an emergent system. There is no one neuron that contains an idea, but it is in the firing of millions of neurons that an idea emerges. Human beings and cultures are emergent systems. Poverty is an emergent system. Those living in poverty exist in an ecosystem that none of them are able to fully recognize or understand. But that system influences them greatly. Brooks highlights a study by Eric Turkheimer from the University of Virginia in which he showed the negative impact of poverty on the IQs of those enmeshed in that ecosystem. But even though Turkheimer spent years of study trying to determine what part of the experience of living in poverty actually caused the detriment to IQs, he was unsuccessful. There was no causal link, even though the total effect of all the variables combined was very clear.

That is the problem with emergent systems: there is no one or two or even three or four things you can point to and say, "Fix that, and the problem will be solved." That does not mean you do nothing. It just means you cannot think of the problem like a clock.

So it is in long-term care. Organizational culture is like a cloud, not a clock. It is an emergent system. There is no one person who exemplifies an institutional culture, but the interactions of all of us who have worked within the institutional system have created this thing called institutional culture. And by its very existence, institutional culture influences us all as well as shapes our behavior. And it has shaped our behavior for generations without anyone planning it or even thinking about it. And as new people come into the system, it changes them as well. Through our work to change that emergent system, however, in a way we are fighting poverty: the impoverishment of the human spirit.

The institutional model of care has taken the good hearts and tireless energy of thousands upon thousands of people who care about elders and crushed them beneath a mountain of rules, regulations, policies, schedules, and routines. It has created a cloud so thick, that those inside it cannot even see the impact it is having on them. But those on the outside can see; they see the cloud and they do not want to breathe its noxious fumes. They say, "I'd rather die than live there." Or "I don't know how you do that work!"

We need a new cloud, a new emergent system, if we want to create something truly sustainable. Leadership must begin by understanding the problem and then focusing on the whole, not just the parts. We need a new pathway to true sustainability, a new way of life, new eyes, new beliefs, new practices, new ways of treating each other, new language, new narrative, and new measures of success—a new cloud that is enduring, that speaks to each of us, and that changes us from within. From that personal transformation emerges a bright new cloud that is a better place to live and work. From inside that cloud, we can change programs and practices and create new artifacts that support the new ecosystem and will be passed down and endure for generations.

The Return from La-La Land

Remember, it's your life. You can live it in La-La Land looking for that one day that your ship will come in. Or you can live each day deliberately.

—David Foster, minister

The early adopters of culture change in long-term care were an amazing group of people who were fearless in their pursuit of an ideal. Armed with little more than a few guiding principles and the hearts of gentle revolutionaries, they took their vision of a better world and worked defiantly within and without their organizations to bring person-centered care to life. There was absolutely no evidence this would work. There were no tools or resources or experience to guide them; no road map to keep them on track and complete uncertainty about the journey. They endured the scowls and mockery from the status quo. They suffered the slings and arrows of naysayers and cynics, all in pursuit of a dream, an ideal.

Through their hard work and indomitable spirit, they have changed the landscape of long-term care. They have brought their ideal into mainstream thought and practice. In Colorado, a full 50% of the state's pay-for-performance add-on reimbursement to the Medicaid daily rates includes person-centered care practices. Every long-term care conference across the country now includes presentations on person-centered care. You cannot even go into a long-term care community now without seeing live-in animal companions. I have been a part of this movement for so long that I remember the days when even that was seen as a radical idea, one over which we had to fight tooth and nail with every state government in the country. In my tenure at The Eden Alternative, I spent the better part of a month ensuring animal rights activists that we would care as much for the animals as we would the people living in our community.

So, we've come a long way, baby. Yet, we have miles and miles to go before we sleep.

FROM REVOLUTION TO EVOLUTION

rev-o-lu-tion \ ˌrevə'lo͞oSHən \ *n* 1. a forcible overthrow of a government or social order in favor of a new system. *syn:* rebellion, revolt, insurrection, mutiny, uprising, riot, rioting, insurgence, seizure of power, coup (d'état)

ev·o·lu·tion \ ˌevə'lo͞oSHən \ *n* 1. the gradual development of something, esp. from a simple to a more complex form. *syn:* development, advancement, growth, rise, progress, expansion, unfolding

The early adopters of person-centered care were revolutionaries. I think we had to see ourselves in this way to sustain our passion and commitment. We had to believe we were overthrowing the current regime (the institutional model of care) and all that was wrong with that system, to find and sustain the energy necessary to make the leap to our ideal of transforming care to be person-centered. We felt we had to uproot the current ruling system and return power to the people (the elders). We banded together in solidarity and spoke of our passion and fervor for the rights of our elders. We battled against the status quo and the restrictive control that was denying our elders and those who cared for them their rights to autonomy and a life worth living. We fought against the plagues of the human spirit and a meaningless existence imposed by institutional thinking and practices that were so ingrained into the current system that nothing less than a total revolution would dislodge them. Revolutionary or transformational change is pro-found. When we think revolutionary change, we envision complete overhaul, renovation, and reconstruction. This type of change is dramatic and often irreversible. From an organizational perspective, revolutionary change reshapes and realigns strategic goals and often leads to radical breakthroughs in beliefs and behaviors.

So a revolution was needed. But revolutions often leave behind some destruction. And there is also danger that the revolutionaries, seeing themselves as having won, will stop growing, thereby exhibiting the hubris and arrogance of conquerors, rather than the humility that leaders need to sustain a movement. Revolutions leave people behind because not every care community has a revolutionary leader. Not everyone is willing to take those kinds of risks. Most people need a road map and some assurance of success before they journey into new territory. Our movement is scrambling to create both so that person-centered care moves beyond the early adopters.

I once heard Maya Angelou say, "The truth is, no one of us can be free until everybody is free" (https://www.youtube.com/watch?v=UxkTd6BFL1o). I believe that is true. Therefore, we must work very hard to make this transformation easier so that all care communities can experience the joy of its success. We must create new tools and resources to help others follow in our footsteps, paving the way so their journey is easier.

Now is the time for the evolution to begin.

Evolutionary change is incremental and takes place gradually, over time. It happens step by step, little by little. The greatest benefit of evolutionary change is that it brings with it all of the practices, behaviors, and advances that are good in the old identity; it builds on the strengths of the organization so that its leaders can imagine going further. Evolution builds on the success of the past to create the future.

A REVOLUTIONARY APPROACH

Piñon Management in Colorado was blessed to have had a revolutionary leader in Jeff Jerebker, an early pioneer of the person-centered care movement. Now semi-retired, Jeff was engaging in culture change and person-centered care in his communities before there was even a term for it. Piñon Management has a reputation for leading the way in a new way. Its managed communities have been at the forefront of innovative practices in a person-centered model of care for more than 30 years. I was both honored and humbled to have been invited by Jeff to work with him. I remain both after 8 years of being a part of an incredible organization that has since evolved into Vivage Senior Living joining with another great organization, Quality Life Management, in 2012.

When I first started in my new position at Piñon Management, I was astounded by the depth of person-centeredness that existed in the organization. It was truly the driving philosophy of the company, a philosophy that had attracted some of the best and most passionate leaders in the business. These leaders had done amazing things. You could walk into any Piñon community and feel the love.

Shortly after my arrival, however, it began to become painfully clear to me that some in our organization perceived a community with a person-centered model of care as a low accountability environment. It seemed to some that if we truly care about our employees, then we would not hold them accountable. In some communities, there was also a deep focus on quality of life; while quality of care and financial outcomes were still good, they were not meeting the highest standards of the organization. It was as if through the revolution from an institutional to person-centered care model, our communities had made a leap so far away from the institution that they forgot to bring the good parts with them.

I came to call this phenomenon La-La Land. The Piñon communities had made the leap away from the institutional model of care, that is true. However, they had leapt so far that they made it all the way to La-La Land. A warm and friendly place to be, La-La Land feels good. No one is ever uncomfortable. We laugh and play and dance all day. And no one ever grows. Because human growth involves pain. And pain is outlawed in La-La Land.

The problem with La-La Land is that it is not sustainable. If we are not growing, we are actually moving backward. No one understood that more than Jeff. He knew that what these incredible leaders had created was in danger of not surviving.

The Piñon communities were blessed with fine administrators who had accomplished amazing things. But they were misguided in believing they were on a sustainable person-centered path. Yes, they had some great outcomes. People were happy. They had accomplished things many other communities struggle to replicate. Yet they were on a collision course with the future. They needed to begin the return from La-La Land to a true caring community where each person has the opportunity to continue to grow.

Jeff also understood that for his communities to continue to grow on the person-centered path, the corporate offices would also need to take a radical path of transformation. Piñon had been undergoing organizational redesign for 3 years prior to my arrival. It had been a painful and highly disruptive journey; many people who wanted to maintain the status quo chose to leave in the process. Still, this amazing leader remained committed to progressive change.

Jeff took us on an extraordinary path of individual and organizational growth that led us back to sustainability. But not just sustainability. Through organizational redesign, including self-managed teams at the corporate offices, he created a context in which each person could be the best he or she could be in the world.

The return from La-La Land would mean that all of our communities would also have to undertake that painful path to becoming sustainable and beautiful. For all of us who worked for Piñon Management, that meant a deeper understanding of what Jeff called "dialectics," which he defined as seemingly opposing forces that, once harmonized, would create something larger and better than the sum of their parts. And they did.

LESSON 20
The Power of the Dialectic

The yin & the yang are opposite forces. Yet, they exist together in the harmony of a perfect orb.

—R. A. Wise, author

Merriam-Webster defines *dialectic* as "a method of examining and discussing opposing ideas in order to find the truth." Jeff Jerebker understood the power of the dialectic, the idea of tension between two opposing forces leading to synthesis. His chosen symbol or logo for his company was the yin yang symbol, a dialectic that reconciles opposites into a unified whole. Jeff knew that things that were seemingly opposing in the old culture actually supported and energized each other in a new culture. In the new culture, we understand that sustainability lies in the harmonizing of these forces to create a dynamic driver for change and truth.

As we learned from the Reality model, our thinking and beliefs drive our behavior. Let us begin our journey back from La-La Land to a truly sustainable person-centered community by changing our thinking and beliefs around some of these dialectics that are preventing our growth.

ACCOUNTABILITY AND CARING

A nurse once said to me, and I quote, "For God's sake! Don't make them do anything. We need them!" All I could do was just stare at her . . . for a long time. At that moment words failed me. It was as if I had entered a parallel universe where people spoke nonsense, but were deadly serious about it. All I could do was walk away, shaking my head, trying to understand what she meant. After a while, I realized that she was speaking from her own fear of not having enough certified nursing assistants (CNAs). At that time, our community was down 14 CNA positions. I could identify with her fear, but her approach to solving the problem was completely wrong.

Had I succumbed to her fear, we would have never achieved a full complement of highly accountable CNAs who worked together to meet the goals of the community and the needs of our residents. In fact, I would venture to say that we would have been like every other nursing home in central Texas at that time—struggling to stay afloat by using 75% agency staff.

What I knew then, and what I continue to drive home to everyone who will stop long enough to listen, is that *a person-centered model of care requires a higher accountability, not a lower one.* That means a higher accountability for everyone. I call it *universal accountability.* Where the institutional model took a few tireless people, made them the only accountable ones, and then worked them to death, the person-centered model holds everyone accountable. Person-centered care is a high-accountability, high-support, low-hierarchy model. To attain this shift, we first need to redefine what accountability is.

REDEFINING ACCOUNTABILITY

One of the problems with accountability is that people have mis-defined what it is. In the institutional model of care, we have equated accountability with threats and punishment (e.g., "If you do that again, I will write you up!"). I have seen personnel folders containing dozens of "write-ups," yet those people continue to work in the community, continue to disregard the write-ups, and continue the behavior. So they get written up again and again and again. I once found an employee folder with fourteen write-ups in it. I asked the director of nursing, "In this community, how many write-ups does each person get?" Her response was, "Oh, all those are for different performance issues." So this one person had committed fourteen infractions so egregious that they merited a written counseling, and he still had a job. How is this considered accountability?

There is a perception or belief that threats and intimidation are the long-term care managers' only vehicles for holding people accountable. Yet, it is obvious the write-ups are not working. They never lead to anything other than another write-up. To "hold accountable" is always something we would rather do unto others than have be done unto us. But even doing unto others brings pause to our hearts when it comes to accountability. Most people, employees and managers alike, think of accountability with trepidation and, therefore, creatively avoid it. Employees avoid accountability because in a fear-based culture they actually choose to disengage; their motivation leaks out of them, like the air out of a punctured tire. Our managers often avoid accountability because it makes them uncomfortable to "hold others accountable." It is often easier to pray the employee leaves or transfer her to another department or a sister community. *Accountability* is the one word in our lives as leaders that needs to be redefined the most.

Merriam-Webster defines *accountability* as "the quality or state of being accountable; *esp.* : an obligation or willingness to accept responsibility or to account for one's actions."

Nowhere in that definition do I see anything about beating people over the head, threatening or intimidating them. Nor do I see anything about falling into fear. For accountability to be universal, employees must be willing to grow and account for their actions, and managers must be willing to support that growth. By avoiding accountability, the manager is actually putting her own comfort needs above the growth needs of her employee. And by using fear and intimidation as the means of holding others accountable, we have created a demotivating context.

Personally, I do not respond well to threats. If you want me to be the best employee I can be, then do not threaten me. It is demeaning and demotivating, and it will cause me to disengage. Threats and intimidation are tactics used by our federal and state governments in regulating our care communities. As managers of those communities, we do not like that. We complain about it all the time, but then we turn around and use the same tactics on our own staff. And then they disengage.

The problem is that we have placed people into the service of the organization, rather than placing the organization in service to the people. Let us look back at the Reality Model. If we have a filter on our belief window that "people are accountable to the organization," then when they fall short of our expectations of them, we get angry and want to punish them. When we put people into service of the organization and then punish them for failing to meet our expectations of that service, we do not create a context for high performance and creativity. Instead, we create disenchantment and fear.

Fear is the most unproductive force in a care community or for that matter any organization. And it runs rampant throughout our care communities. We have become a fear-based profession. We have perpetuated a punitive, fear-based culture that begins in Washington, D.C., and flows all the way down to the charge nurse on the evening shift. There are certainly many things in our work that could drive fear into our hearts. There are a lot of people looking to find fault with us. State and federal regulators wander our halls, searching for our mistakes. Plaintiffs' attorneys lurk in the bushes outside our windows, just waiting for a human error they can capitalize upon. Some corporate consultants are still pointing out everything that is wrong with us. And so managers walk around trying to find the mistakes before anyone else does and punish the people who make them. Fear is present and accounted for most days in a care community. But we must not succumb to that fear and pass it on to our employees (Pascotto, Goddard, & Gallwey, 2010).

When something goes wrong in our care community, as leaders, we need to change our default response. Stop the automatic habitual response of trying to name, blame, and shame; instead, go to the place of *compassion and curiosity.* Go to compassion rather than blame. Then get curious about what factors may have influenced the problem.

Psychologist Alice Isen found that positive moods facilitate creative problem solving and that negative emotions, such as fear and sadness, can lead to brain activity and thought patterns that are detrimental to creative, productive work. These include the avoidance of risk, difficulty remembering and planning, and rational decision-making.

So creating a fear-based punitive culture is actually preventing our employees from being the creative problem solvers we want them to be. But even more than that, what is it doing to them physically? *What happens to us, as human beings, when we are in a constant state of stress?*

The stress response in humans evolved as a means of protection for us. In the short term, stress can help us. It can actually save our lives. But in the long run, when stress is chronic, it can kill us. Thea Singer (2012), in an article published in *Psychology Today*, helps us better understand why long-term, chronic, and repeated stress is so harmful to us. Singer notes that when the brain receives a stress stimulus (say, you come face to face with a tiger), it sends a signal through the sympathetic nervous system to the adrenal glands to release a hormone called epinephrine. We know this hormone as adrenaline. Some people enjoy an adrenaline rush. But what is adrenaline actually doing to your body? Adrenaline dilates the bronchial tubes so that more oxygen can get through and charge your heart. That enables more blood to push through. Adrenaline also dilates the blood vessels leaving your heart so more oxygen can get to your brain and your muscles. Now, when your brain tells your muscles "RUN!," you are ready.

While that is happening, another hormone, norepinephrine, begins to gush from your nerve endings. That hormone's job is to compress the veins that are returning blood to your heart, creating a stronger surge in the heart. That blood then exits the heart with greater force. At the same time, norepinephrine also constricts the veins to your skin in case you are injured, so the blood flow out of your body will be slower.

Next comes the doozy: the adrenals then secrete another hormone, cortisol. Cortisol is a pretty cool hormone. It is the reason you can get out of bed in the morning. Cortisol mobilizes the energy stored in your cells. On normal days, it ebbs and flows with your circadian rhythm, so you have more in the morning when you need it to get going and less at night when you go to bed. Having the right amount of cortisol in your body is critical to good health. But cortisol does some things to you to help you during that stress response. It elevates your blood pressure. It actually shuts down some of your nonessential functions during times of stress, like your reproductive system or your immune system (Bennington, n.d.). You do not need to be trying to reproduce or worry about catching a cold if a tiger is chasing you. These responses to cortisol are meant to be short-lived, just long enough for you to outrun that tiger.

The prefrontal cortex, the most evolved brain region, is where conscious, rational thinking occurs. It also houses the Rider, our self-discipline. It is the brain region that is most sensitive to the detrimental effects of stress exposure. Even quite mild acute uncontrollable stress can cause a rapid and dramatic loss of prefrontal cognitive abilities; more prolonged stress exposure causes architectural changes in prefrontal dendrites, the message receptors at the end of brain cells (Arnsten, 2009). Indeed, high levels of cortisol over a long period of time can induce decreases in memory and can cause "dendrites in the hippocampus to wither." When they stop working, so does your brain (Singer, 2012).

The evidence is clear: prolonged stress is not good for your health or the health of your residents or employees. Stanford University neurobiologist Robert Sapolsky says it best: "Our goal isn't a life without stress. The idea is to have the right amount of stress" (Singer, 2012).

But it gets worse. The kind of stress that never lets up, that many who work in care communities experience daily, can become chronic. Bruce McEwen of Rockefeller University calls that kind of stress "toxic stress." He says, "Things are coming at you left and right and you can't keep up with them." McEwen warns us that with toxic stress there is a kind of "learned helplessness" in which we stop trying to cope because we lose hope. He states, "The more threatened you feel, the less capable you feel, and the worse your physiology is going to be as a result" (Singer, 2012).

Do you have a lot of call offs? Does your staff get sick a lot? Are your absenteeism levels high? You could blame it on the fact that people who work in care communities work in close proximity to many contagions. You might even blame it on the lack of work ethic among your staff. Or you might look at the stress levels in your community. Toxic stress levels can kill people.

Our role as leaders is not to create more fear or even to buy in to the fear. Our role is to calm the fear, and that begins with changing the way we think about and understand accountability. We must help each person who works in our community redefine accountability, so that it becomes a productive force in our organizations, not a destructive force. When we put the organization into the service of our employees, then we can begin to see accountability through a new filter:

ACCOUNTABILITY = GROWTH

GROWTH = CARING

The idea that if I truly care for my employees, I will not hold them accountable is simply wrong. If it were true that accountability and caring were opposite forces, then how would parents ever hold their children accountable? When we truly care for someone, we help the person to grow. And growth involves high expectations, education, and encouragement, not threats and punishment.

The desire to matter, to make a difference, and to excel are basic human drivers. When we redefine accountability as growth, we change the context of our organizations. We begin to draw on those human motivators to unleash the power of each individual we serve. To make this shift, you first have to believe that people want to do a good job. You then need to understand that if they are not doing a good job, then there is a context problem. As formal leaders, we control the context.

Plenty of scientific research supports the belief that human beings have an innate desire to contribute to, succeed at, or master our work. Yet managers tend to believe this is not true. As behavioral economist Dan Ariely (2013) states, "We tend to have this incredibly simplistic view of why people work and what the labor market looks like." Ariely provides evidence that we are also driven by meaningful work, by others' acknowledgement, and by the amount of effort we have put in: the harder the task is, the prouder we are.

People do not shun hard work. Hard work brings feelings of pride and accomplishment. But for hard work to become meaningful and rewarding, formal leaders must remove the barriers and the fear so that each person can reach his or her highest potential. That requires formal leaders to first hold themselves accountable, ensuring there is nothing in the context that is preventing the employee from being accountable. When you have given an employee everything she needs to be successful and have held yourself accountable first, yet she is still not growing, your only option is to change the context in a new way. The story that follows illustrates this kind of accountability and was told to me by an administrator.

A Story of Accountability

We had a young CNA who became frustrated one day with a resident. She walked into the hallway, and in front of other staff and residents shouted, "I hate this f___ing place!" Of course, this came back to me very quickly. I interviewed a few people and documented that many had heard her comment. I asked her to come meet with me. When she arrived, I asked her if she could please tell me what happened. I also asked her permission to write down what she was telling me. She said that was alright. I picked up my pen and tried to capture some of her exact words as she proceeded to go on a rant! She told me how awful the resident was and how demanding he was and that all he did was complain and bitch no matter how hard she tried. And nothing ever satisfied him. When she calmed down, I asked her if I could read back to her some of her own words. She agreed. As I read back her words, she sat quietly. When I finished, I said to her, "Wow, it is not hard to see that you are just not happy here. I want you to be happy. You spend too many hours at your job to be miserable. What do you love to do?" She responded, more softly now, "I love horses." I then said to her, with sincerity, because I truly cared for her, "I think that you will not be happy until you are living your passion. So I am going to let you go and find it. I want to hear from you in a month that you have found a job working with horses." As she signed her termination papers, she wrote, "Thank you. I am going to find work doing something I love." You see, accountability does not mean belittling or demeaning people. It means truly caring for people. (York, personal communication, 2012)

A leader understands that if someone is not growing with you, the only way you can continue to care for that person is to move them to another leader with whom, hopefully, they will continue to grow. But even terminating someone does not have to become a hostile act that leaves the person feeling diminished. It should be an act of compassion and caring.

ACCOUNTABILITY SURVEY

At Vivage Senior Living, we created an Accountability Survey as a tool that administrators, managers, or team leaders can use to hold themselves accountable first and to better understand account- ability as caring. Before a person-centered leader takes any kind of disciplinary action or terminates a team member, he or she must complete the survey to ensure everything in his or her power has been done to help a team member grow. If the leader responds no to any of the questions, he or she must address that specific account- ability factor before any disciplinary action is taken. Once the leader has held him/herself accountable and it becomes clear that the team member is not taking 100% responsibility, then the only means to help the team member grow is through disciplinary action, up to and including termination. The leader must also seek the wisdom and input of his or her mentor before making these decisions. In the process of holding a team member accountable, the leader must model our organization's Code of Ethics at all times.

I have seen the two extremes of accountability: On the one hand, managers who never hold anyone accountable. On the other hand, managers who use punishment and threats in an effort to hold someone accountable. Neither of these approaches is leadership behavior that is person-centered. True person-centered leaders use accountability as a tool for growth and development, both for themselves and others. To do that, we must first redefine what accountability is and in doing so create a context in which each person is motivated to be her best. The dialectic of accountability and caring, when harmonized, is the path to unequaled performance in yourself and all of your employees.

Accountability Survey

1. Have I clearly communicated my expectations to my team member?
2. Am I certain that the team member understands my expectations?
3. Is there something in the system, policy, procedure, or environment that is preventing my team member from meeting my expectations?
4. Have I given my team member the proper training, resources, and support to meet my expectations?
5. Have I listened to my team member's reasons for his/her inability to meet my expectations?
6. Have I clearly documented my team member's reasons?
7. Have I eliminated those reasons or barriers for my team member, if it is within my control to correct?
8. If it is a barrier in his/her personal life, have I offered the opportunity for personal leave or referred him/her to our employee assistance program until that barrier is removed?
9. Is this disciplinary action what is best for our residents?
10. Is it fair to everyone?
11. Is it consistent with other decisions I have made?
12. Am I certain this is not the place where my team member will continue to grow?
13. Have I documented my team member's actions that have led to a disciplinary action?
14. Have I consulted my mentor for his/her wisdom?
15. Have I consulted with our Human Resources department?
16. Having made this decision, will I be able to support it in the future?

QUALITY OF LIFE AND QUALITY OF CARE

The institutional model of care focused on quality of care while neglecting quality of life. This model took 100 infirm elders, put them in a large, institutional, hospital-like building and then assigned 100 people to attend to the needs of their human bodies, yet only two people to attend to the needs of their human spirits. Quality of care has always been the sovereign in post-acute care, just as it is in acute care. The attempts to harmonize these two seemingly opposing forces through the culture change movement have caused many definitive battles. Talk to anyone who has been a part of this movement for any amount of time and they will tell you that one of the most significant challenges they have faced is "convincing" the nurses to take this journey.

There is a misperception that if we focus on quality of life, quality of care will suffer. And if we are honest with ourselves, there are times when it has. The mantra of person-centered care is that when we focus on quality of life, quality of care improves. And it should. But that has not always been the case.

Person-centered care is not throwing the baby out with the bathwater. It is not giving up all of the progress we have made in improving care over the last 40 years so that our residents can tiptoe through the tulips. It is not a diminishment of the importance or focus on quality of care. It is an evolution. It is because of the last 40 years of improving the quality of care that we can begin to imagine meeting the needs of the human spirit as well as the human body.

One can experience quality of care without experiencing quality of life. We see that every day in institutional "zero-deficiency" nursing homes. They do everything "by the book." They dot their i's and cross their t's. And the quality of "care" is excellent. Yet, there's a cold lifelessness that permeates the building. People have checked out.

However, the converse is not true. I contend that you cannot experience quality of life without experiencing quality of care. The challenge for us in care communities is to prevent the lives of our elders from being centered around medical treatment and quality of care. We cannot ignore medical treatment, but we can put it backstage, supporting a human life, not as the star of the show. The elder is the star of her own show, directing her own life as much as possible.

So a focus on quality of life must include a focus on quality of care. It is only through the marriage of the two that we find true person-centered care. Through that marriage, we will spawn an even higher accountability as care communities. That is the aspiration of WELL-BEING for all. Well-being is the unity of quality of care and quality of life. It is the highest measure of success in a human community. But approaching well-being begins with harmonizing the dialectic of quality of care and quality of life. (I delve more deeply into the concept of well-being in redefining our measures of success in Lesson 24.)

MISSION AND MONEY

Somehow along the person-centered journey in our quest to do the right thing, we adopted a righteous disregard about profit. And we are a for-profit company! Maybe that is why this happened. If we had been not-for-profit, the mantra of "no money, no mission" might have been drilled into us. But we were a for-profit, mission-driven company. The mission was alive and well, but we forgot the money part. It just was not a focus.

Most of our homes were profitable. Most were more than 90% occupied. That helped. But our accounts payable were growing, our cash flow was down, and our budgets were out of line. In La-La Land, money does not matter. But in this world, it does. Without it, we cannot sustain our mission.

Money is not the root of all evil. The verse from the King James version of the Bible goes: *"For the love of money is the root of all evil: which while some coveted after, they have erred from the faith, and pierced themselves through with many sorrows"* (Timothy 6:10 King James Version). Money is not evil, the love of money is. I actually prefer the Mark Twain (1905) version: *"The lack of money is the root of all evil."*

Who knows this better than people who work in long-term care, a chronically underfunded system? When money is put toward the mission, it is a good thing. And because we are chronically underfunded, we must be good stewards of our money. We do not have any to waste. That is not scarcity mentality; that is just the facts. We have to watch our pennies.

Person-centered leaders teach everyone in their organization about the benefits of making a profit and how that profit sustains the organization, provides for improvements that benefit the elders, and allows for benefits to staff. Mission and money in a person-centered model are best friends. They rely on each other.

DOING AND TEACHING

I remember the first Piñon Forum I attended. I was actually stunned to discover for the first time from an insider's view that there still existed this huge divide and mistrust between the communities and the corporate offices. Maybe huge is an overstatement, but it was certainly obvious and, at the least, detrimental to our goals of creating an interdependent community with a spirit of oneness. The culture of "us and them," no matter where you find it, is a destructive force to community building.

The punitive culture, top-down hierarchy, and robust chain of command in long-term care has perpetuated this divide between people who work in the same organization. There was a perception in some of our communities that our corporate consultants, most of whom previously worked in a care community, now participated in what my friend David Farrell so affectionately calls "drive-by consulting" (Farrell, Brady, & Frank, 2011, p. 250).

We can trace this divide back to a misdefinition of accountability as punishment and threats instead of growth. People who used to be directors of nursing (DONs) or social workers or activity directors or business office managers in a care community (the doers), and who were very good at their jobs, were "promoted" to the corporate offices, where they are now expected to know how to be a coach and a consultant and a servant leader (the teachers). Their roles demanded a shift from doing to teaching, two completely different skill sets. None of them were given training on how to coach or teach. Yet, now their success depended on the performance of others. This is a formula for trouble that is perpetuated throughout almost every long-term care company.

THE EVIL-DOERS AND THE WHITE KNIGHTS?

So my encounter on this beautiful day during the forum in Colorado was eye-opening. Many of the people who worked in Piñon managed communities saw their corporate consultants as threats, "evil-doers," rather than as resources—until they had an opening in a critical position in their community. Then, they expected these consultants to act as "white knights" and come to the rescue of the care community, filling the slot until a replacement could be hired. The minute that person walked out the door and returned to their role as corporate consultant, they magically transformed back into an evil-doer!

What we needed, beyond a complete redefining of accountability, was the harmonizing of doing and teaching. Our consultants needed to be taught to make the shift from doer to teacher, not enabler. They needed an understanding that what they *do* now is to *teach*.

Some of the most successful administrators in our organization, however, recognized the value of having teachers and mentors, experts in a certain area who would come to their community, not to rescue or punish, but to grow capacity in others. They built strong relationships with their consultants and appreciated them. And guess what happened? The consultants wanted to go to those communities. They wanted to help grow others. And when they returned to the corporate offices, they did not start gossiping and bad-mouthing the people in those communities, as the drive-by consultants are prone to do.

Be warned: this pull back to the old culture of thinking and behavior for consultants is extremely hard to overcome. In times of stress, we return to old patterns of behavior. But through the development of self-directed functional and cross-functional teams at the corporate offices, the education of our consultants as leaders, and the expectations that they will be in service to our communities, there was a shift in the illusionary divide between corporate and community staff. A spirit of oneness began to replace the old divide. These leaders still have to remind themselves at times not to fall into community bashing and instead talk about how they can serve each community, but the change has been palpable.

EMPIRICAL DATA AND STORY

In La-La Land, we know we are doing a great job because everyone is happy and smiling. It feels warm and welcoming. You hear administrators saying things like, "I feel like we are making progress on reducing our overtime." Having a caring community and relying on empirical data to support your case for the effectiveness of a person-centered model of care are not inconsistent.

Warmth and welcoming and happiness are wonderful indicators. Anecdotal data in the form of stories open people's hearts so that they can open their minds to a new way. The culture change movement has survived decades on these kinds of heart-warming, culture change stories. They tug at our heartstrings, and research shows that emotion and motivation are tightly linked (Brooks, 2011).

In fact, studies have shown that people who have experienced illness or injury have damaged the emotional part of their brain, the limbic system (Brooks, 2011). Emotion involves the entire nervous system, of course. But two parts of the nervous system are especially significant: the limbic system and the autonomic nervous system. The limbic system is a complex set of structures that lies on both sides of the thalamus, just under the cerebrum. It includes the hypothalamus, the hippocampus, the amygdala, and several other nearby areas. It appears to be primarily responsible for our emotional life and has a lot to do with the formation of memories. People who have suffered damage to these parts of the brain have still been able to rationalize, plan, and conduct analytical thinking, but they are unable to make a decision and move forward on that thinking. Again, motivation and emotion are linked. If you want to move people to action, you need to "find the feeling." Stories are a powerful way to do that (Brooks, 2011).

But administrators and other community coordinators cannot know if they are making progress without hard empirical data. Data and storytelling are a dialectic that, once harmonized, can bring powerful transformation to your community. In a person-centered community, data are not kept a secret and are shared freely with all stakeholders, which creates the opportunity for everyone to participate in process improvement.

With today's technology, we have a greater access to information and data than ever before. The question becomes, then, what are we doing with it? Do we make a pile on our desks that we bring to the quality assurance meeting once a month? Do we look at the data, have a meeting to report on it, and then do nothing else with it? Or are we using the data daily in our practice as a person-centered administrator?

Empirical data are an important tool in creating a caring community and is like any other tool—if we never use it, it is not really a tool. Person-centered administrators say that they "own" the data and information and "share" it with everyone. This means that they take responsibility for the quality of information that is used within the community for process improvement and that they share information with all stakeholders. They recognize that information is power and when everyone has information, everyone can contribute to the success of the organization. They believe in and practice transparency.

Being transparent is hard to capture in just one sentence. It is about sharing all of the information the receiver wants or needs, not just the information that the sender is willing to share. It is about putting all facts on the table, even when some facts are uncomfortable to receive. It is about being honest and open about what actions are taken, by whom, and on what grounds. It is about enabling people to have open and honest conversations, thereby creating mutual understanding. It is about removing any barriers that hinder people from accessing the information they could need to be better at their jobs. It is about making people and their skills, knowledge, and ideas visible and accessible to all of their colleagues.

By engaging all stakeholders in process improvement, the action items and plans you develop will have a better chance of success. You can sit in your office all day reviewing data and coming up with action plans, but will you have all of the information? Will you have the most creative ideas? To be truly person-centered, you not only share data and information, but you also engage others in creating the improvement plans.

Through our Neighborhood Guide program and the development of self-managed neighborhood teams, in some Vivage's communities you will find hands-on staff (including nurses, CNAs, housekeepers, activity or social services staff, even residents and families) in the huddle that follows an incident or accident. They conduct a root-cause analysis with all of the information available, decide on a plan to prevent the incident or accident from happening again, and make that action plan a part of the care plan. This creates a context for highly creative solutions to come forth. The hands-on staff, who did not participate in process improvement in the old culture, are now "child-like" in their problem solving. By that I mean that they are not just going through the motions, trying to satisfy the state requirements for a new intervention, as many of our managers have been reduced to doing. No, these care partners are invigorated with the creative energy and ideas that managers, stale to the process, can no longer envision because their automatic brains have not kicked in. These care partners are not entrapped by the old paradigm of what a fall intervention (or other solution to a problem) can be. They bring much-needed new eyes and new ideas to process improvement.

Without empirical data to show these teams how their work is impacting quality outcomes for the residents, I doubt we could inspire them to continue this practice. "I feel like Mr. Smith isn't falling as much as he used to do" is not as compelling as "We have reduced Mr. Smith's falls by 50% in the last month." However, hearing a CNA tell the story of Mr. Smith, whose family brought him to stay with us because he was falling at home but who is not falling as much because we have reduced his medications by 75% and he's even speaking again, is also very compelling. So marrying the powerful stories with the empirical data creates sustainability, ownership, and growth.

CHANGE AND SUCCESS

"If it ain't broke, don't fix it!"—a cliché that is no longer valid. In an environment where change is occurring exponentially, if you are not changing, you'll be left behind. As I look across the landscape of the culture change movement, it is easy to see early adopters who made great strides initially, but somehow got stuck. They stopped growing. Organizations joining the movement after them stood on their shoulders. They came into the movement later, when more information and knowledge was available, and their starting place was way ahead of where the early adopters began. So their journeys were taking them deeper into person-centered care, while the early adopters were being left behind, basking in their forgotten glory.

The belief, "We are successful, we don't need to stretch ourselves," is dangerous. The saying goes, "Good is the enemy of great." So the cliché should be, "If it ain't broke, break it!" And keep breaking it. Success lies in continued growth.

HUMILITY

What our early adopters needed was a large dose of humility. Humility is one of the most important traits for a leader, especially during times of great change. The minute you start thinking that you have made it is the minute you start losing ground.

The empirical research on humility shows that this trait has great value. Humility has been linked with better academic performance as well as excellence in leadership. Humble people have better social relationships, avoid deception in their social interactions, and tend to be forgiving, grateful, and cooperative. A set of studies also shows that humility is a consistent predictor of generosity. People who are humble tend to be more generous with both their time and their money. Generosity then lends itself to an abundance mentality, which you will recall from Lesson 16 is an important leadership characteristic (Exline & Hill, 2012).

CHANGE IS THE CONSTANT

Dr. Bill Thomas told me something early in my journey that has stuck with me for years. He said, "All great people are chronically dissatisfied." Not such a happy thought! But it has taken on deep meaning for me as I enter into my twenty-first year in the person-centered care movement. Now I understand that he was saying great leaders always see the gap between the way things are and the way they ought to be. And there will always be a gap. They understand that success is dependent upon change, constant change, enduring change.

Jeff Jerebker taught me a Buddhist saying, "Change is the constant," meaning that the only constant in the world is that change will happen. Everything is changing. If we look at long-term care, in particular the last 30 to 40 years, we see how this is true.

> Buddhism holds that everything is in constant flux. Thus the question is whether we are to accept change passively and be swept away by it or whether we are to take the lead and create positive changes on our own initiative. While conservatism and self-protection might be likened to winter, night, and death, the spirit of pioneering and attempting to realize ideals evokes images of spring, morning, and birth. (Daisaku Ikeda, in Higgins & Bergman, 2011, p. 31)

So the return from La-La Land must also include the enlightenment that in a rapidly changing world, success in the past does not guarantee success in the future. We must continually be engaged in our own rebirth. You could have the best person-centered care model in the world today and not be in business tomorrow if you stop growing. Change and success are tightly woven together. Do not try to separate them.

There are many dialectics in the world of long-term care that, when harmonized, begin to shape a new and exciting world. These are just a few of the more predominant ones. Watch for these as you continue your journey of leadership and enlightenment. This concept of seemingly opposite or contrary forces that are actually interconnected is an important one for us as leaders who are in pursuit of an interdependent community in which a spirit of oneness fosters cooperation and creativity. Many interacting forces can form a dynamic system in which the whole is greater than the parts. That is the path to sustainable change. That is creating a new cloud.

Now that we have an understanding of the problem of creating sustainable person-centered care, we can begin to understand how to solve it. Let us use the science of leadership to elevate the art of leadership.

We learned through the Reality Model that our brains take our beliefs and create unconscious paradigms that drive our behavior in an effort to meet our needs. So to change behavior, our own as well as others', we must shift our beliefs. We must change the filters on our belief windows that are creating behaviors that keep us mired in institutional behavior. For that kind of behavior is surely not meeting our needs or our desires of creating a caring community.

As I stated in Lesson 9, we all hold millions of beliefs. We have big beliefs, like moral and ethical beliefs, as well as small beliefs that drive our behavior. I once had a boss who believed that his employees should arrive at work at 8:00 a.m. and not leave until 5:00 p.m. He did not really care or even monitor what they did between those hours or how productive they were. He just wanted them there during those hours. That belief then led him to look at his watch if someone came in a few minutes late and to write people up if they left work early. It did not matter to him that his employees had personal lives, or car trouble, or traffic problems, or were not morning people. There was no important meeting they would miss if they did not arrive on time or left early. Other people were not waiting on them to arrive. What kind of context for performance do you think that created?

If you guessed that his employees resented this kind of top-down authority, you would be right. If you guessed that his employees underperformed, you would be right again. They showed up on time. They worked until 5:00 p.m., but they did just enough to get by. Now, if he could have justified why getting there on time and staying until the last minute truly mattered, it would have been a different story. But in this case, it was just his belief, a belief that held no justification. His micromanagement created a context and a belief by his staff that he did not trust them. Therefore, they were demotivated and responded in kind.

Who knows where that belief came from. He might not even be able to tell us. But it was firmly planted on his belief window and had gone unexamined by him for years. What are some of the beliefs that you have firmly planted onto your belief window that have gone unexamined? You will never know all of them, but the next time someone that you are leading exhibits a behavior that you do not like or understand, you best look in the mirror first.

This journey from institution to caring community is a challenging one, indeed. It is not for sissies. It is going to challenge you to shift your own beliefs to create a new context or a new "cloud." In the next chapter, I describe some of the shifts in beliefs that will support your journey toward a caring community. It will be up to you, though, to make the shifts.

CHAPTER 6

Solving the Problem

Shifting Our Beliefs

LESSON 21
From Sheepherder to Shepherd

If you change the belief first, changing the action is easier.

—Peter McWilliams, author

Have you ever seen sheepherder dogs work to keep all of the sheep going in the right direction? They dash back and forth, nipping at the heels of the sheep, tongues hanging out, panting furiously. Do you ever feel like that? If so, it is time to make a shift in your beliefs and behaviors. Hopefully, the lessons in this chapter will help you stop nipping at heels and get out in front like a shepherd and lead.

BECOMING A COACH AND FACILITATOR

The institutional model would have us believe that there are two subspecies of Homo sapiens: management and staff, as if managers and hands-on staff have taken separate and divergent evolutionary paths. Nothing could be further from the truth. We are all the same. We have the same needs. We are motivated by the same factors. We have the same hurts and disappointments and the same delights and joys. But the institutional model taught us that we are different. It taught us that we, the managers, are the only accountable ones. So, managers direct and monitor. We tell our staff what to do, when to do it, how to do it, and then stand over them and make sure they do it! And if they do not do it, we punish them.

I had spoken to a group of administrators outside of our company. I asked them to write down their greatest problem, the thing that was keeping them up at night. I was surprised to read the first card:

"My staff won't break down the boxes before putting them into the dumpster unless someone is watching them."

I could not help it—before my rational mind could kick in and stop me, I fell right back into the sarcasm I learned from my southern roots. I asked this administrator if he had hired someone to watch them to make sure they did it. Then I suggested he should just make it part of his rounds each day to go out and break down the boxes himself, since his employees were so incompetent.

Then I realized the error of my outburst. Fortunately for me, we all live in a culture where sarcasm, the lowest form of humor, is acceptable and even lauded. So everyone laughed. But I then shook myself out of my automatic responses and recognized that this was a teaching moment. I asked the group, "Why do we want staff to break down the boxes? Why is it important?" Of course, I got the typical institutional response, "Because if the dumpster isn't closed, the state [read: enemy] will give us a deficiency."

And the staff know that. But we know that knowledge does not change behavior. Although the staff want to do well on surveys, it is not a real motivator for them. Is there something else in the system or context that is driving this behavior (not breaking down the boxes)? I told the group to stop using the state as a threat to their staff. Threats do not motivate. And when we use the state as a threat to try to control behavior, we are creating a very dangerous situation. If the state is the enemy, then every time they enter your community, you have created a context for high stress, which shuts down the rational, thinking brain.

So I asked again, "Why do we and the state want the staff to break down the boxes? Why is it important?" Finally, one person said, "Because if the dumpsters are left open, it could bring unwanted pests that might bring disease that could be harmful to our residents or staff." Bingo!

There is the motivator, the common denominator that we all share. None of us wants to do anything that would harm our residents or each other. So, facilitate a discussion with staff about the *real* reason it is important to break down the boxes: not because we might get into trouble, but because we have a responsibility to our residents and each other. Change their belief.

But there is still the problem of context; that is, why is the staff not breaking down the boxes before putting them in the dumpster? The best way I know to learn why is to ask them: "What are the barriers to doing what is best for the residents?" Sit down and talk to them. Listen to their challenges. Quit assuming that they are just lazy or do not want to do a good job. Trust that the solution to the problem is there waiting to be discovered. Then ask them what you could change that would help them be able to break down the boxes. Then make that happen. Or, hire someone to watch over them and make sure it happens. Those are your choices.

We have to stop being problem solvers and start becoming coaches and facilitators of a group process. We have to let go of our ego needs of being the one with all of the answers and instead create an environment in which all stakeholders together help solve the problem. *Ask questions, do not give answers.* Your job as a formal leader is to educate and explore, then bring resources to the solutions your staff find. Do not forget to congratulate them for being such great problem solvers. Your job now is to "coach" and "facilitate." Those are two of the new skills you will need to become a shepherd.

Coaching is the art of helping others discover the answers for themselves. It requires skills in listening without judgment, paraphrasing, and asking open-ended questions to help the person or team you are coaching work through the issue and find a solution. It requires a very strong rider muscle and patience. Coaching takes more time than telling someone what to do. However, the investment in the growth and development of your employee pays off exponentially down the road in your own well-being as well as theirs.

Facilitation of the group process is another shepherd skill that is critical for person-centered leaders. The word *facilitate* means to make easier. The goal of facilitation is to make the group process easier. Facilitators guide the group process toward its goals. As we move away from the institutional model of care, we move away from individual decision making and toward a group or team process. Understanding team development and having the skills to facilitate the development of high-functioning teams will become one of the most important skills for leaders. Coincidentally, both coaching and facilitation require the coach and the facilitator to subsume their own egos, letting go of the need to be the decision maker. It is ironic that the very trait that made you a formal leader, your ego-drive, is the one that you must now diminish to master the art of leadership.

Part of the journey to a sustainable person-centered model of care is the opportunity for everyone in the organization to grow together. There are enough people outside our profession who want to find fault with us. We do not have to find fault with each other. We do need to continue on a path of improvement and growth. That journey is much more fun if we take it together.

THINK COMMUNITY INSTEAD OF INSTITUTION

If you have been working in the institutional model for any time, even just a few months, you have put some pretty strange filters on your belief window. If you have worked there for years, you are now mired in institutional thinking. Shifting beliefs requires a team of people who are in a high-trust relationship and can challenge each other. The institution has its claws embedded into every aspect of our thinking. We must challenge each other to think differently. One of the ways you can begin to do this is to challenge everything you are about to do by asking, "Is this the way we would do this at home?" You will be surprised by how often you will find that the answer is a resounding no.

In mentoring the nursing home administrator at the Green House project in Loveland, Colorado, I once came across a situation that illustrates this point. The institution is a part of us, and we bring institutional thinking with us, even when the entire environment and organizational design has been changed. In this case, the NHA, with the best of intentions, created a worse problem while trying to solve a problem.

There was some conflict going on between the shahbazim in one of the houses and one of the nurses who worked in the evenings. The shahbazim felt that this nurse was being disrespectful of them and their time by coming in and "demanding" that they get her vital signs on a resident while they were in the middle of other tasks. They resented this treatment and expressed that to John, the NHA, who was their guide. John then told the nurses in all of the houses that the shahbazim would no longer be getting them vital signs. The nurses would have to do it themselves. Problem solved. Hardly.

I discovered that this decision had been made because I had been meeting with the nurses and the NHA to discuss the barriers they had to working within their budgeted hours. I had asked for them to come up with some solutions to help us remain in budget. One of the nurses then told me that it would help if the shahbazim could get vitals on their elders. John immediately "confessed" that he had made this decision already and apologized for it. As a group, we talked about the need for a common respect and a willingness on everyone's part to help each other. The nurses have an obligation to build a good relationship with the shahbazim so that they will want to help them. This can be done by helping the shahbazim when they have time. Then the shahbazim will be much more likely to reciprocate.

The NHA and I talked after the meeting about the decision he had made and its unintended consequences. How many times do we make decisions that have unintended consequences? In this case, the NHA's institutional response to interpersonal conflict was to create a policy that everyone had to live by, rather than effectively managing the conflict and coaching the nurse in how to be respectful of the shahbazim. That one decision drove a deeper wedge between nurses and shahbazim, and it ended up costing the community precious dollars. It was not the only reason nurses were working over budgeted hours, but it certainly contributed. This decision also meant we lost the nurse who created the conflict in the first place, because the conflict was never resolved. And it meant that all of the other nurses were paying dues for her behavior. Wow!

I asked the NHA what he would have done if he had thought community instead of institution. He responded that he would have brought the shahbazim and the nurse together to work through the issue and to discover how they might work together respectfully in the future. He understood how trying to solve human problems by coming up with another policy that all were forced to live by was never the answer. That is institutional thinking. And it only creates more problems and resentment.

DEVELOPMENTAL AGING

Institutions in the United States were created to house and care for our frail elders based on the societal beliefs we have adopted about aging. If you grew up in the United States, unless you were part of a subculture that held its own beliefs about aging, it is likely you hold the societal belief that aging is about decline. All you need do is to turn on the television or open a magazine to have these beliefs reinforced daily. Truth be told, we are all ageist. Try this test. For the next 24 hours, become aware of every ageist remark, image, joke, or thought that you come across. You will be astounded. Even old people are ageist.

There is a multi-billion dollar industry based on these beliefs that aging is bad and only about decline. According to Transparency Market Research, the global anti-aging market is expected to be worth more than $190 billion by 2019 (Transparency Market Research, 2015).

Think about that for a minute. Anti-aging. Against aging. People will be spending $190 billion each year by 2019 to try to stop aging. There is such a dread of becoming old that people will endure and pay for high-risk treatments to not look old. I answered my door one day, and my neighbor was standing on the porch. Her face looked like she had been through a fire. It was red and swollen and peeling. She was hardly recognizable. I gasped and asked her what happened. She told me that she had volunteered to test a new kind of anti-aging treatment that uses a laser to literally blister the outer layer of skin on your face off so that it can be peeled off. She said she had been in misery for days and that she actually looked better that day than she had for the last 3 days. I asked her why she had done it. She told me it was vanity. She did not want to look old. I told her my wrinkles do not hurt. And until they do, I am not going to let someone blast my face off (Transparency Market Research, 2015).

In his book, *What Are Old People For: How Elders Will Save the World*, Dr. Bill Thomas gives us a different view of aging. His view is not of aging as decline, but as a continued stage of development. As we age, our bodies may start to decline, but we continue to grow and develop as human beings, intellectually, emotionally, and spiritually.

I have personally found this to be true. I wrote this book at the age of 66, and it is much evolved from the first book I wrote on leadership 10 years ago. And prior to that first book, I did not know enough to write a book on leadership. So at the same time that my knees seem to be declining, I have continued to grow and develop as a human being.

So why is this shift in beliefs from the declinist's view of aging to a developmental view important for a person-centered community? The entire system of long-term care in the United States is based upon the declinist's view of aging. That view led us to create "God's Waiting Room." It defined our roles as people who mitigate the negative aspects of aging. It positioned us as people who try to take something that is very bad and make it a little better for the moment, knowing that it is a losing battle. With that kind of mission, it is surprising that we can even get ourselves out of bed in the morning. It is not surprising that there are not enough people who want to do this work. By shifting the belief of aging to developmental aging, let us paint a new mission for ourselves and our staff.

Our elders are not diminished or broken adults. They serve a noble purpose in our society. They are our greatest teachers. They teach us how to live as human beings. They teach us about compassion, forgiveness, patience, and tolerance. Because we have lost the wisdom of our elders, our society is suffering. Our children are suffering. As a society, we are becoming less and less compassionate and patient and forgiving and tolerant every day.

When we embrace the belief that our elders continue to grow, we begin to see our role differently. Our role is to grow the most positive elderhood possible as well as to grow the sacred art of caregiving. Our elders will save the world through us—we, who know them well and benefit every day from the lessons they share with us. That is a mission worthy of our attention, passion, and energy. When we shift our own beliefs about aging and those we care for, we elevate the meaning and purpose of the work we do. That is a reason to get up in the morning. That is a reason you can use to attract and retain great people. When our elders have great value, our work has great value. Make that shift in the beliefs of your employees. Help them see how valuable our elders are.

COMPLAINTS

The institutional model taught us that complaints are something to avoid at all costs. We have made it one measure of our success to have no complaints. I want to shift that belief for you right now. Instead, define success, in one part, by not having any complaint surveys, because you should have lots of complaints coming to you and not the state.

In a human community where people feel safe and heard, they will complain. That is how we behave as humans. Think about your own family and friends. Do you ever hear any complaints from them? Do you ever complain?

Not having any customer or staff complaints is a dangerous thing. If you do not have any complaints, that means people either are afraid of retribution or have given up hope that anything will ever change. Neither is a context for growth. People complain when they feel they will be heard and that the complaining will make a difference. They complain when they feel that it is safe to complain and that they will not be blamed or labeled for being a complainer.

We must begin to shift our beliefs about complaints. Complaints are good! They are gifts. When someone complains to you, they are telling you that they trust you. They are giving you an opportunity to make it right, because they believe in you. So you should thank them for the gift and then go about making it right. Certainly you do not want the same complaints happening over and over. That means you were not listening or you have not gotten to the root cause of the problem.

I know at the Green Houses in Loveland, Colorado, we have many people who complain. The staff there was a little worried once about our annual survey because they were fielding complaints on a daily basis. I told them not to worry. I knew that we were addressing those complaints. No, things were not perfect, but we were working on it. We acknowledged people each time they came to us with a complaint, and we told them everything we were doing to try to improve. When the state came for their visit, they did not receive any complaints from the elders. The elders told them that everything was wonderful. They loved it there!

I believe in my heart that because we created a caring community where everyone felt safe to complain, those who complained protected us from the "outsiders." They did not feel the need to tell the state our community issues. They did not need to share our "dirty laundry." In a truly caring community, we take care of each other and we trust each other; and we complain to each other, but not to outsiders.

Teach everyone in your community that complaints are gifts and should be received with gratitude. Teach everyone how to handle a complaint and to work toward resolving it. That is how a community acts.

In the next three lessons, I discuss shifts we need to make in our beliefs around work ethic and motivation, empowerment, and our measures of success to move away from institutional thinking and behavior toward creating a sustainable caring community.

A New View of Motivation

To succeed, you need to find something to hold on to, something to motivate you, something to inspire you.

—Tony Dorsett, former NFL football player

I have often heard that it is a manager's job to motivate their employees. I disagree with that belief. I believe that people motivate themselves, and it is a leader's job to create a context in which each person can find his or her own motivation.

What context motivates people to be their best? What does it look like? What does it feel like? What components of human motivation must be present in this context?

We are going to explore those questions with some interesting research on motivation, but first I want to share some enlightenment that I came across in a workshop presentation by Barbara Frank in 2016 at a quality symposium. Barbara is one of those culture change pioneers who I can count on to always bring me new leadership perspectives. I enjoy learning from her. In this seminar, she shared information from two different sources that I hope will begin to shift some of your beliefs regarding human motivation. I know they have been eye-opening for me.

The first source is *Bridges Out of Poverty: Strategies for Professionals and Communities* (Payne & DeVol, 2006), a tool designed for service providers and businesses whose work connects them with those living in poverty. The authors offer a deeper understanding of the challenges and strengths of people living in poverty to help in partnering with them to create opportunities for success. The authors present a picture of the middle class experience, which is characterized by stability, predictability, and safety. Middle class people believe they can achieve through their hard work the things in life that can improve their lives. They also have the ability to anticipate and problem solve most bumps they find in the road. Our society and our workplaces expect workers to have stability in their lives and the ability to plan for and cope with unusual circumstances in their lives. In fact, most workplaces have very little tolerance for those who cannot do this. The poverty experience, however, is different from the middle class experience of stability and safety. If you live in poverty, life is falling apart all the time, and you do not have the resources to fix it. When you live in poverty, life is unstable and uncertain. You rely on relationships with family and friends to help bring some stability, but you live in the "tyranny of the moment," waiting for the next crisis to bring it all crashing down. And without resources to anticipate and handle problems, a crisis could be a broken-down car, a sick child, or a sick mother who cares for your child. It could be having enough money to buy food or gas or to go to the doctor.

Bridges Out of Poverty also discusses the role of language and story, specifically the "word gap" between children from low-income homes and their more economically advantaged peers. Based on research from Risley and Hart (1995), between the ages of 1 and 3, children from different socioeconomic cohorts have very different experiences regarding exposure to language. Children in the welfare class are exposed to about 10 million words during these ages in comparison to working class children, who are exposed to 20 million words, and the children of the professional working class, who are exposed to 30 million words. Even more important are the messages they are receiving through those words. If you were raised in the welfare class, for every affirming thing said to you, you received two messages that discounted you. In the worker class, this is reversed: you get two "Attaboy" for every "What the hell's wrong with you?" And if you were lucky enough to be raised by professional parents, you were given five encouraging words for every discouraging word.

The second source is research commissioned by the Kansas Association of Homes and Services for the Aging. The study was led by Mary Lescoe-Long and Michael Long, who looked at what affected staff retention, satisfaction, and performance in skilled nursing homes in Kansas (Lescoe-Long & Long, 1998). To better understand, they divided the staff into three cohorts: paraprofessionals (CNAs), front-line supervisors (nurses), and managers/department heads. Their research found three factors at play in the retention, satisfaction, and performance of these cohorts: "predisposing circumstances," "organizational reinforcers," and "interpersonal reinforcers." There were circumstances in people's lives that influenced them to behave in certain ways, and the researchers found that organizational and interpersonal factors reinforced that behavior.

When they looked at predisposing circumstances, the researchers found significant differences among the three cohorts. Now, there are certainly exceptions, but this was the abundance of indicators they had found. The paraprofessionals, or CNAs, largely came from severely economically challenged backgrounds; the frontline managers, or nurses, largely came from what Lescoe-Long and Long called "lower middle class" families; and the managers and department heads backgrounds were largely classified as "middle class."

Because of their predisposed circumstances, the paraprofessionals lacked a causal link between their personal effort and their success. In other words, they were unable to see a connection between how hard they worked and how their lives might improve. This is probably because they had seen their parents work hard all their lives but remain impoverished. They themselves were working hard and still lived on the edge. In contrast, the nurses' personal backgrounds gave them what they called a "bootstrap link" between their effort and their success. They believed that they had pulled themselves up by their bootstraps and so can everyone else. The department managers had a robust sense of self-confidence and personal causality in that they believed they could greatly improve their personal circumstances through their hard work. There is clearly a conflict in beliefs among the three different cohorts, and we already know how beliefs drive behavior.

When Lescoe-Long and Long looked at the effect of predisposing circumstances on the different cohorts' motivation to learn and grow, they found that the paraprofessionals were used to external factors controlling their lives. Their learning needs were great but very fragile. Their motivation to learn could be undermined by the smallest problems. The nurses were used to relying on their own problem-solving skills and were not as controlled by external forces. They took pride in having worked hard to earn respect. The department managers had experience in using their own abilities to produce good results and were in search of opportunities to learn and grow.

The paraprofessionals lived in the tyranny of the moment, which had such a great effect on them that it undermined and overwhelmed any willingness they may have had to learn. They could not attend an in-service if they were worried about getting to the power company to pay their bill before the power was cut off. They could not think about going to nursing school to work their way out of poverty if they could not even make it through the pay period with enough food for their families. The tyranny of the moment destroyed any motivation they may have had for growth and development.

How do predisposed circumstances affect job training and preparedness? The research showed the paraprofessionals found an incongruity between how their jobs were depicted in training and their actual jobs. And many of them were unprepared for the challenges of the residents they were responsible for caring for. The nurses, especially LPNs, were not prepared for managing people. Even department managers had little training in how to manage people, especially people with different skills and circumstances.

The research also showed that there were circumstances, or context, within the skilled nursing homes that reinforced these disconnects among the different cohorts. CNAs had very little decision-making power and were told what to do by nurses. Can you see how a lack of any decision-making authority would undermine and reinforce the belief that a CNA may have about the uselessness of trying to learn and grow? Can you also see how the nurses, without management training, would respond to a lack of initiation on the part of CNAs by being more controlling of them in deciding and delegating what they should be doing? This leads to resentment on both sides, but most especially on the part of the nurses toward the CNAs ("I shouldn't have to tell you what to do! Just do your job!").

The researchers concluded that the reinforcers in the interpersonal relationships among the cohorts present as a lack of mutual empathy. The paraprofessionals held a belief that their supervisors did not understand what their lives were like. The nurses misunderstood the source of the CNAs' behavior and came to the wrong conclusions about the causes of that behavior, which grew resentment. The department managers may have been sympathetic to the circumstances of the paraprofessionals, but they were not empathetic because they did not understand the circumstances.

Lescoe-Long and Long's research also showed there was a mutual lack of interpersonal skills across the three cohorts. The paraprofessionals were likely to respond to stressful situations with "conflict generating" responses. The nurses' education gave them good communication skills for communicating with residents but not with staff. The department managers showed good interpersonal skills until they came across someone who did not have those. Then they were in trouble.

I share this research in the hopes that you can begin to shift some of your beliefs about your employees' behavior. Maybe what you perceive as a lack of motivation, just maybe, is because of the context in which they live. The tyranny of the moment and the beliefs that were passed on to them in those 10 million words they heard at an early age are driving some of the behaviors that frustrate the nurses and the department managers. Perhaps if we act with empathy instead of sympathy, we can ask ourselves, "What can we do as leaders to create a context in which each person can have stability and success and experience well-being?"

As managers and middle managers we must shift our beliefs to better understand motivation. How can we overcome the impact of the tyranny of the moment to create a context for motivation among our employees? I have a few clues about that. At a time when nursing and CNA staffing is in short supply in most communities, at Vivage Senior Living we have a waiting list for staff in our Green House homes in Loveland, Colorado. Less than 2 years ago, we went into a suburban market in Loveland that was already experiencing a shortage of nurses and CNAs. We pulled out of that market almost 60 CNAs and 20 licensed nurses, RNs, and LPNs. And if you want to work at the Green House homes at Mirasol, you have to be hired as PRN and wait for an opening.

How did we do this? We created a context that motivates people to stay. And, yes, you can do the same, even in a traditional physical plant environment with a 50-year-old building. In the next two lessons, I tell you how. Right now, I want you to begin to shift your beliefs around motivation. STOP, do not jump to those next two lessons. Remember, shifting beliefs comes first. It is time to shift yours.

———————

At Vivage, we had an administrator complain to our Human Resources Director that he was losing staff because he was not paying them enough. However, in exit interviews with staff, the HR Director found only one person out of the six had left for more money. Money and benefits are important motivators. People need to make money to live in these modern times. In order to attract competent staff, you must know the market rates for the positions in your community and be comparable. Our HR department has done a remarkable job of analyzing market rates for each job position and determining the low, middle, and high ranges our communities use as guides in setting wages. Yet, we still have nursing home administrators (NHAs) who believe it is about the money.

You do not have to be the employer offering the highest wages in your market area, but you do need to be in the mid-range to continue to attract new employees. Once those external, or extrinsic, motivators are comparable, what can you do, as a leader, to create that context for people to stay?

In his book, *Drive: The Surprising Truth About What Motivates Us,* Daniel Pink helps us see motivation through a new lens. Drawing on research on human behavior, Pink suggests that when it comes to motivation, there is a gap between what science knows and what business does. Pink uses the analogy of motivation as operating systems. In Motivation 1.0, early in human history, Pink talks about our biological motivators of hunger, thirst, and sex. These motivators were not much different from other animals. This system of motivation served us until it did not. When we had to cooperate with others to survive when more complex social systems were built, we needed an upgrade in our motivational system. Pink describes this upgraded system as Motivation 2.0, our extrinsic, or external, motivators. This is when we began responding to rewards and punishments in our environment, what Pink calls "carrots and sticks."

Businesses have been using Motivation 2.0 for a very long time. Pink states,

> Humans have uniquely mastered this operating system and channeled this drive to develop everything from contract law to convenience stores. . . . Motivation 2.0 assumes humans aren't much more than horses; dangle a carrot in front of our noses or hit us with a sharper stick and we will go in the right direction. (Pink, 2009, p. 18)

In long-term care, we rely heavily on the sticks versus the carrots.

Pink also discusses current research that reveals Motivation 2.0 is very unreliable. Even carrots can sometimes be demotivating. We have already learned about the detriments of using sticks as a motivating force. Relying heavily on rewards can create a "goals-only" focus that could create a narrowed focus, unethical behavior, increased risk taking, decreased cooperation, and decreased intrinsic motivation. I have actually seen this happen in organizations that use very high bonus structures for their NHAs. This does not mean we stop rewarding people, just that we be careful about how we use rewards so that they do not create these problems.

Pink suggests that we need a new motivational operating system he calls Motivation 3.0, which is based on our intrinsic, or internal, drivers. Since the middle of the 20th century, scientists have been studying this third drive. Businesses have not caught up with this new understanding. Pink suggests that Motivation 2.0 is so ingrained in us, we do not even think about it. It has become a habit and is a part of our automatic brains.

Motivation 3.0 suggests that we are driven by much more than our biological needs and external forces. In 1960, Douglas McGregor, an MIT management professor, published *The Human Side of Enterprise*, in which he suggested company managers were operating from faulty assumptions about human behavior. He offered a different view:

- Humans take as much interest in their work as they do in their rest or play.

- Creativity and ingenuity are widely distributed in the population.

- Under proper conditions people will seek responsibility.

Do you share these beliefs? If so, what are the proper conditions in which people will seek responsibility? Pink suggests that Motivation 3.0 has the answers in drawing upon three intrinsic motivators:

- Autonomy
- Mastery
- Purpose

Human beings are born with a need for autonomy, the need to direct their own lives. Anyone who has ever had small children knows this to be true. It delights me to no end to watch my 2-year-old granddaughter assert her autonomy over her parents. That innate need does not disappear or diminish as we grow older. The institutional model conspires to change that default setting in all but a very few employees. Person-centered leaders, however, aspire to meet that need in their employees.

Pink defines mastery as "becoming better at something that matters." He tells us that "Motivation 2.0 requires compliance, while Motivation 3.0 demands engagement. Only engagement can produce mastery" (Pink, 2009, p. 111). In the institutional model, mastery becomes our definition of mastery, not our employees' definition. We define mastery as compliance with tasks, schedules, routines, and regulations. The only path to growth in the institutional model is through a "career ladder." Those who want to remain in their chosen position are not provided with a path to mastery or the opportunity to grow.

Human beings crave purpose. It is in our nature to seek out opportunities to be a part of a cause greater than ourselves. The institutional model takes the noble hearts of caring people and crushes them, stripping away the meaning and purpose in their work. Then we wonder why people leave or why we have high absenteeism.

So, why does the Green House project in Loveland have a waiting list for staff? The model builds upon the three intrinsic motivators. One of the core values of the Green House model is "empowered staff." The organizational design creates empowered teams who work together and expands the roles and authority of CNAs as managers of the houses. It flattens the hierarchy. It provides the hands-on staff with opportunities to grow in their own positions without having to become a nurse (or the nurses to become the DONs). And it restores the meaning and purpose to their work. One of the craziest ideas Dr. Bill Thomas has ever had, if you ask some people, is having chosen the name *shahbazim* (Persian for *king's falcons*) for the universal workers in the Green House homes. But Bill has a reason for everything he does when creating new models of care, and this may be one of his smartest. He found a new identity for the CNAs that has no preconceived values or assumptions tied to it. From that new identity, shahbazim all over this country are growing that identity to its mastery.

I do not care what your physical plant looks like. I do not care how old it is. You can achieve Motivation 3.0 in your care community by establishing person-centered leadership practices and creating a context in which intrinsic motivators are present. I know. I have done it. And I have seen other person-centered leaders accomplish the same. Stop focusing on what you do not have and focus on what you do have. You have the opportunity through your leadership to create a community where people want to live and want to work, a place where every person motivates themselves because of the opportunity for autonomy, mastery, and purpose. To create that place, you must also shift your beliefs about empowerment, which we'll cover next.

LESSON 23
Empowerment as a Function of Leadership

When things go wrong in your command, start searching for the reason in increasingly large circles around your own desk.

—General Bruce Clarke, U.S. Army

Since W. Edwards Deming completely transformed Japanese industry following World War II, companies have been adopting employee empowerment and team-based organizational design in increasing numbers. In almost every industry, employee empowerment and the development of self-managed teams is the norm. Every industry, that is, except long-term care.

Why are so many companies adopting this type of organizational design and leadership? The results are undeniable. In a 1995 article in *Quality Digest*, Ron Williams shared a *Business Week* report that characterized self-managed work teams as "30 to 50 percent more productive than their conventional counterparts." *Business Week* listed the following as examples of companies that had attributed much of their success to the development of self-managed work teams (Williams, 1995):

- AT&T: Increased the quality of its operator service by 12%.

- Federal Express: Cut service errors by 13%.

- Johnson & Johnson: Achieved inventory reductions of $6 million.

- Shenandoah Life Insurance: Cut staffing needs, saving $200,000 per year, while handling a 33% greater volume of work.

- 3M's Hutchinson facility: Increased production gains by 300%.

In his article, Williams reported that in a survey of 500 companies, top managers identified the following outcomes as reasons for their decisions to move toward this new way of working (are any of them appealing to you?):

- improved quality, productivity, and service
- greater flexibility
- reduced operating costs
- faster response to technological change
- fewer, simpler job classifications
- better response to workers' values
- increased employee commitment to the organization
- enhanced ability to attract and retain the best people

We learned from Daniel Pink in the previous lesson about the intrinsic motivators of autonomy, mastery, and purpose. Employee empowerment creates a context for all of those to exist.

So why have our long-term care communities not embraced this type of organizational design and leadership more fully? The person-centered care model, The Eden Alternative® philosophy, and the Green House® model all espouse employee empowerment through self-managed teams. Yet, when I first arrived at Piñon Management in 2008, I found that none of our communities had fully embraced the concept or made strides toward this new way of working.

There certainly have been some brave souls who have ventured toward these types of teams. In their book, *In Pursuit of the Sunbeam*, Steve Shields and LaVrene Norton discuss empowerment through their Household Model™. The Green House Project has been using empowered teams for more than 10 years. Very few communities, however, have maintained their traditional physical environment and achieved true cross-functional self-managed teams.

I have come to understand that many people in our field, although eager, are reluctant to try this new organizational model because the barriers seem too high. First, they just do not know how. I have also found that many people do not truly understand what *empowerment* means. There have been these ill-fated attempts at "self-scheduling" that put people off to the idea. The consequences of a failed attempt at empowerment in our work could be devastating. Then there is the fear of failure and/or loss of control that plague many managers in long-term care. In this lesson, I want to help you better understand empowerment so that you can begin to shift your beliefs around it, for it is truly the path to creating sustainable person-centered care.

EMPOWERMENT IS NOT . . .

We are going to use the Socratic method of defining something by first defining what it is not. I find this method of understanding very useful. So, what is empowerment not?

Abdication

Abdication is formally relinquishing your authority. When leaders empower teams to have decision-making authority over their work, it does not absolve the leader from her own responsibilities.

Think of a parent who is helping her teenager to be empowered to drive a car. The parent does not toss the teenager the keys to the car and walk away. No, the parent is right there sitting beside the teenager, risking her own life! The parent is responsible for teaching and training the child how to be a good driver. The parent is responsible for setting the parameters or limits for the child. The parent provides the child with knowledge and information he needs to be a successful driver. The parent is right there when the child messes up, providing a supportive environment in which he can learn from his mistakes.

The same is true in care communities. Every self-managed team needs people who serve as guides who help them grow. These guides do not relinquish their own authority or accountability to the team. They are there every day making sure empowerment conditions are in place. Empowerment is a function of leadership. It requires the leader's ongoing participation in shifting authority and accountability out of the formal ruling structure and into the team.

Anarchy

Anarchy is a state of disorder due to the absence or nonrecognition of authority. Empowerment is not anarchy! Just because the team is empowered, it does not mean they get to make decisions selfishly, without parameters. It does not mean they can make

decisions based on their emotions rather than the ethical principles that guide all decision making in your organization.

Empowerment is by its very definition the moving of both
authority and accountability together out of the formal hierarchy
and into the team. You cannot separate the two. People try to separate them all the time. Let us go back to our teenager. Teens want
authority. They do not want the accountability that comes with it.
But parents understand you cannot have one without the other.
Managers, however, expect their employees to be accountable
without giving them the authority that comes with it.

Think of the lyrics to that old song: "Love and marriage, love
and marriage; go together like a horse and carriage. This I tell you
brother, you can't have one without the other." When it comes to
authority and accountability, this still holds. So parents tell their
teenagers, "Show me some good grades, and we will talk about
learning to drive." And if the kid messes up, the parent holds him
accountable. Certainly how we hold our children accountable will
look different than how we hold a team accountable. Leaders hold
a team accountable by ensuring that the team members hold each
other accountable. They do not punish the team or "ground" them.
They coach the team through a root-cause analysis of the problem
and then through problem solving and action planning to minimize the risk of it happening again.

Self-managed teams hold the authority, so they also hold the
accountability. The manager must ensure that accountability is
present and accounted for every day. Anarchy is not a good context for a care community.

Assumed

Empowerment should never be assumed. It does not matter how
long your teams have been functioning. Just because you trained
the team, told them they were an empowered team, and put them
together in one neighborhood or household does not mean they
are empowered or even a team.

People who have worked in traditional long-term care may
take a while to trust enough to take on decision-making authority. They may still believe that they will be punished if they make
the wrong decision. Often they will not even tell you if they need
something, such as more information and resources. Remember

the Parkview story and the story of the "Farmer and the Hoe-maker" I shared in earlier lessons? Never assume that just because you have "empowered" your employee that they will act empowered. Guides of self-managed teams are present daily, asking the team if they have everything they need to be successful.

Regular and consistent team meetings must flush out issues that may be impeding the team's progress. One of the biggest mistakes I see guides making is that because the team is functioning well, they think they do not need to meet. Without that consistent opportunity to address team issues, the team will soon start taking short cuts or get engaged in unresolved conflict that will threaten the team. Remember, in our world we are growing teams across departments and shifts. We are growing teams who may not see each other consistently without that meeting. Do not assume everything is going well. Hold team meetings regularly to find out. Ideally, new teams should meet weekly or at least biweekly. Once training is complete and there has not been any turnover, and the team has become a performing team, then you can try moving the meetings to monthly. But should trouble arise, do not be afraid to go back to more frequent team meetings.

Advisement

Empowerment is not advisement. I have heard managers say, "Oh, yeah! I am an empowering leader. I go and get input from the team before I make a decision." That is just getting input. You still maintain all of the decision-making authority. And if you get input and then do what you want to do and ignore the input, you foster resentment and resistance. Empowerment moves the decision-making authority out of the current ruling structure and into the team.

What are you empowering the team to do? A self-managed team is empowered to make decisions over their TASKS (what they do), TIME (when they do it), TEAM (who they do it with), and TECHNIQUE (how they do it). In our work, the self-managed teams are empowered to provide excellent customer service without usurping the decision-making authority of the residents.

I was coaching an NHA from Alaska who was working to grow self-managed teams. She emailed me with a problem she ran into with one of her teams. While the NHA was out of town, an elder wanted to change rooms to another neighborhood. Staff would not let her and met with the elder and her son. They told the elder that she could not move because she was a fall risk and her current neighborhood had more staff. They claimed more people walking by her door somehow protected her. They also claimed that she would lose the strong relationships she had in her current neighborhood if she moved. They resorted to all kinds of institutional excuses in an effort to control the elder. I do not blame them. Those same practices have been tried on staff for years.

The elder responded that she would be in the same facility and could still see the staff. When the NHA told the staff that they could not tell the resident she could not move, they responded with, "See, we knew we weren't really empowered." So it is very important that, first, each team has more than one guide, and, second, the team be given the full scope of their decision-making authority. Authority over tasks, time, team, and technique does not mean they are empowered to direct the elders. Team empowerment does not make the team a monarchy.

All of the team's decision-making authority is still within parameters, just as your own decision-making has parameters. One of the guide's jobs is to make sure everyone on the team understands the parameters. In Chapter 7, where I discuss changing the context, I give you tools to help you set clear parameters around decision making, including a Principles of Ethical Decision Making (Lesson 31), but also a Code of Ethics. You are not empowering the team to decide your benefit package or your budget. You may give them the budget as a decision-making parameter, but their decision-making authority is limited, just as yours is.

Assignment

Empowerment is not assignment, better known as delegation. (I needed to stick with the alliteration.) Assignment is when you ask someone to do a part of your job. It is an extremely important management technique. Managers delegate duties or tasks to others all the time, but do not confuse delegation with empowerment. With delegation, you are asking for help. You are in no way moving decision-making authority or accountability to that person.

I write more about team empowerment in Lesson 26 on organizational redesign. Here, I want you to shift your beliefs about empowerment and help you begin to see it as a function of leadership that requires the leader's ongoing participation. Empowerment is not something you do *to* people. It is something you do *with* people.

In our environment, we are empowering teams of people to work together to improve the lives of our residents. We are not empowering individuals to do whatever they want to do. We are not making a bunch of kings and queens. We are creating an opportunity for a group of people to work as a high-functioning team to meet the goals of the community, in alignment with the values and priorities of the organization.

I have seen some resistance to employee empowerment from department managers who perceive it as a threat to their jobs. Nothing could be further from the truth. We still need those managers. We just need them to shift their roles from being the decision makers to being the guides for self-managed teams. Breaking down that resistance begins with shifting their beliefs about empowerment.

Now that we have an understanding of what empowerment is not, let us define what it is for our care communities: *Empowerment is the moving of both authority and accountability out of the traditional departmental hierarchy into a cross-functional team committed to meeting the individual needs and desires of the people they serve.*

I want to share one last insight about empowerment. Empowerment cannot fail. It is a proven means of unleashing the creative energy and potential in each person. What can fail is the leader. Refer back to General Clarke's quote at the beginning of this lesson (*"When things go wrong in your command, start searching for the reason in increasingly large circles around your own desk."*) Empowerment fails when the leader fails.

A word of caution. If you are going to undertake the important and valuable work of empowering teams in your care community, then do it right. You cannot and must not ever "try empowerment." It is not a game. It is serious business that must not be taken lightly or without due diligence. And once you begin, you never stop. When something goes wrong, look in the mirror and ask yourself, "What did I fail to give the team to help them become successful?" As Deming told the Japanese, 85% of the problems in a company are caused by the managers.

In my own company, this failure of leadership occurred around empowerment. Our leadership and operational resource teams, the formal leaders at Vivage, have always (at least as long as I have been there) been empowered to make decisions about what conferences we and our team members attend. We have been trusted to know where our growth needs are as well as how we can promote the company through conference participation. We pride ourselves on being a "learning and growing" organization. At a team meeting, one of our owners announced that he was instituting a new policy. Without explanation or reason, he decided that we would now each be limited to one conference per year, and we had to get approval. He then had our controller pass out a new form that stated this policy and required that we estimate the cost of attending a conference and plead our case as to why we should attend. You could have heard a pin drop in the room. The meetings after the meeting ran rampant. Trust had been broken, and all for naught.

I found out later that a number of people had attended a very expensive conference in California at a luxury resort. In response to that problem, the policy was implemented that basically said to team members, "We don't trust you." The lessons from this one decision are huge for leaders who want to engage in empowerment. What our leadership failed to do was give us the parameters around conferences. There was no budget. There were no recommended conferences or conferences that were off limits. There was nothing to help us determine how many conferences to attend. Empowerment did not fail. Leadership failed.

Once a problem arose due to leadership's failure, the decision-making authority of the team members was jerked back. Do not ever do that. When you do, you break trust that is difficult to regain. Besides, rarely do we solve problems with policies. That is institutional thinking and practice. The solution to the problem of conference attendance was to give the team parameters and to facilitate a discussion about the best way to make conference decisions going forward. Then trust that the team wants to do a good job. Trust that they will adopt the practices the team decides upon. If the parameters change, go back to the team. If the problem persists, go back to the team. Have them conduct a root-cause analysis and come up with a better plan of action. And keep going back until it is no longer a problem. Then go on to the next problem. That is good leadership, and that is true empowerment.

I do need to give my owners the credit they deserve. Once this breach of empowerment was brought to their attention, they were able to see the error of their ways. They created new parameters to guide us in our decision making about conference attendance. Being a leader does not mean you never make a mistake. It means when you do, you are not too prideful to correct your mistake. We will all make rash judgments in the heat of the moment. When we do, we apologize, learn from the mistake, and move forward.

Redefining Our Measures of Success

One measure of your success will be the degree to which you build up others who work with you. While building up others, you will build up yourself.

—James E. Casey, founder of UPS

How do we measure success in long-term care? We actually have many ways to measure success. We have clinical indicators, financial indicators, human resource indicators, customer and employee satisfaction surveys, regulatory outcomes, and a lack of complaints. The Centers for Medicaid & Medicare Services has now given us the Five-Star measure. And the Patient Protection and Affordable Care Act of 2010 has given us hospital readmissions as an indicator of success.

All of these measures, with the exception of lack of complaints, can translate to a person-centered model of success measurements. They are all important, and they are all linked. Maintaining excellent clinical outcomes is an imperative for avoiding regulatory Hell. Whether you work in a for-profit or not-for-profit community, having good financial outcomes is important and vital to both good clinical and human resource outcomes. Without good human resource outcomes, you cannot provide good care or have financial or regulatory success. Love it or hate it, the Five-Star rating is an important measure for success. It is how customers and other healthcare providers rate us. And if you are sending a lot of people back to the hospital, you may need to look at your clinical systems.

They are all good measures, but will they help you to grow a sustainable, caring community? What is the measure of success for a caring community? How will we know when we have attained it? How will we know we have not just put wings on a caterpillar and called it a butterfly?

Those were the questions we asked ourselves in 2004 as pioneers in person-centered care. We understood that the current measures of success would not get us where we wanted to go. Today there are plenty of Five-Star nursing homes that are still institutions and not true care communities. There are the pretenders of culture change: homes that have all of the pretty trappings, but elders are still languishing unnecessarily beneath a pile of policies and procedures designed to maximize efficiencies. There are "zero-deficiency" homes, where employees do as they are told and never disrupt the status quo.

Pablo Picasso once said, "When we love a woman, we don't start measuring her limbs." So, what do we measure? To help answer this question and to develop tools for measuring true person-centered care, The Eden Alternative assembled a group of experienced person-centered researchers, educators, and early adopters. With assistance from the Jefferson Area Board of Aging in Charlottesville, Virginia, the group met over 3 days to discuss this important topic.

To address the topic, the group had to shift their beliefs from a declinist's view of aging to one of old age as another stage of growth and development in human life. They had to think in terms of how a community supports a life versus an institution. They determined that the ultimate outcome of a life worth living is well-being and that the ultimate outcome of a caring community is the well-being of the people who lived, worked, and visited there. They believed that improving the well-being of residents would enhance the well-being of the community itself.

Then the question became, "What is well-being?" The group identified seven domains of well-being. Before you read further, write down everything you need in your life to experience well-being. You can have as many or as few things on your list as you want. Do not leave anything out. Now, look at the list of well-being domains that follows, as identified by the group. Try to fit the things on your list into at least one of the domains. Some of the things on your list may fit into more than one domain, but see if you can fit them into at least one.

- Identity

- Connectedness

- Security

- Autonomy

- Meaning

- Growth

- Joy

Do you have anything left over? I have done this exercise all over the country with many different groups. Only a few times have I had anyone with leftover well-being needs. Usually it is "good health." Other members of the group then help that person see how "good health" might fit into several of the domains, including Security, Identity, Autonomy, or Growth, to name a few.

However, for the people living in our care communities, good health might not be attainable. This is why it is not a domain of well-being. This model does not presume what we consider "good health" to be a precursor for well-being. The premise here is that everyone can and should have the opportunity to experience well-being despite any physical or mental incapacity or health challenge they might experience. That said, the model also presumes that those incapacities and challenges have been identified and are being addressed according to current best practices.

Let us explore each of the domains a bit further.

Identity is being well-known, having a personhood, being an individual, having a history, being whole. No one can exist without an identity. How many of you have attended a resident's funeral, only to learn something about the person you never knew? That is because the institutional model strips our elders' identities away, leaving them virtually unknown. It reduces their identity to what is wrong with them. They are known by a diagnosis or a room number or payor source. The institutional model also reduces the individual identities of our employees to a job position. The model denies people the opportunity to be known in their own community.

Connectedness is the state of being alive and engaged, of belonging. We are connected to other living beings, to the larger living world, and to each other. We are connected to the past and the future, to our possessions, and to a place we call home. Without those connections, we become susceptible to the plagues of the human spirit as well as the body.

Security is the freedom from doubt and uncertainty. It is feeling safe, certain, and assured. It comes with having privacy, dignity, and respect as well as from being deeply known and knowing others in your community. Person-centered communities have consistent staff who build relationships with residents so they can feel secure. Staff honor residents' rights to privacy and autonomy, which creates a sense of security.

Autonomy is the freedom to direct your own life, to have self-determination and immunity from the arbitrary exercise of authority over you. Autonomy also means you have a choice, in what you eat, what you do, and where you go. Denying autonomy invites sympathy, pity, or even invasive paternalism.

Meaning is what we hold sacred. Stripping the meaning away from something one holds sacred is profane. Meaning is hope and heart. It is value and purpose. Meaning is essential to human health.

Growth is development and enrichment, unfolding, expanding, and evolving. Elders and staff have growth needs that must be attended to. When we stop growing and learning, we stop living fully.

Joy is beyond happiness. Happiness is fleeting. One can be happy one minute and sad the next. Joy is a state of being. It is the ultimate outcome of a human life. When one's needs for identity, connectedness, security, autonomy, growth, and meaning have been met, one can live in a state of joy (Fox et al., 2005).

Remembering the Reality Model, everything we do is in an attempt to meet these well-being needs. Sometimes those attempts are misguided because of an ill-founded filter on our belief window. If we can shift beliefs, then our behavior will shift to meet our needs.

But what happens when we feel our well-being needs are not being met? How do *you* respond when you feel your needs are not met? Do you cry? Do you sulk? Do you yell? Do you run away? Do you strike out? Do you drink or take drugs? If you respond with any of these behaviors, has anyone ever suggested you take some Haldol? Why do we think our elders require medication when they are expressing an unmet need? Why do we label them a "behavior problem" and ask a doctor to order a psychotropic medication to control the behavior? Instead, hopefully you become self-reflective and try to change your behavior to get your needs met. Doing so will shift your belief about and understanding of expressions of unmet needs so that when faced with any of these responses from a resident, you will ask, "What need are we not meeting in this person?"

I encourage you to read my friend Dr. Al Power's two seminal works, *Dementia Beyond Drugs* and *Dementia Beyond Disease*. Through his work, Dr. Power is helping many in care communities around the world begin to shift their beliefs about dementia and their role in caring for those living with it. His work has spawned a revolution in dementia care. You should be a part of it. The next time one of your residents expresses an unmet need, instead of blaming it on the resident or a disease process, put the onus on yourself. Consider the domains of well-being and try to discover which needs are not being met. Then adjust your behavior and the behavior of the care partners to meet those needs. Change the context, and the behavior will stop.

Do you think your employees ever feel that their needs are not being met? What do you do when an employee exhibits an expression of an unmet need? Do you respond in kind? Do you threaten or punish the person? Or do you ask, "What need are we not meeting in this person?" In a truly caring community, we do not look to place blame on someone who is struggling; we adjust our own behavior to meet the person's needs.

I want to share with you another African custom that stems from a cultural belief of Ubuntu, the belief that we are all connected by a universal bond across all humanity:

> In this African tribe, when someone does something harmful, they take the person to the center of the village where the whole tribe comes and surrounds him. For two days, they will say to the man all the good things that he has done. The tribe believes that each human being comes into the world as good. Each one of us only desiring safety, love, peace and happiness. But sometimes, in the pursuit of these things, people make mistakes. The community

sees those mistakes as a cry for help. They unite then to lift him, to reconnect him with his true nature, to remind him who he really is, until he fully remembers the truth of which he had been temporarily disconnected: "I am good."

Shikoba Nabajyotisaikia!

Nabajyotisaikia *is a compliment used in South Africa and means:* *"I respect you, I cherish you. You matter to me." In response, people say shikoba, which is: "So, I exist for you."* (Sunnubian, 2014)

I often wonder what would happen if an entire leadership team and care partners were to surround an employee who was expressing an unmet need and tell the person all of the good things she has done. Would that create a context where each person can experience well-being? Try it and see.

The domains of well-being are not just for creating a better world for your residents. They also can be used to create a better world for your staff, the residents' family members, the staff's family members, and you. When we no longer believe that we are successful if we have met the institution model's measures of success, we can stretch ourselves further. We can begin to recognize that success is only found in meeting the well-being needs of all in our community.

Thinking and Behavior Matrix for Person-Centered Leaders

You are free to create your own paradigms instead of simply accepting those presented to you by others.

—Russell Eric Dobda, author

You are free to create your own paradigms. Or you can accept the gift I am about to share with you. We each have many filters on our belief window. These filters have been placed there by the fact that we have worked within the context of an institutional model. These beliefs have given us one way of seeing the world. From these beliefs, our behaviors have been shaped. We need to shift our thinking to shift our behaviors.

There are far too many institutional model beliefs for me to mention in one book. I run into new ones every day. For example, a very influential person in my organization once told me that he did not want to encourage relationships between consultants and the communities they served. His belief was that if the consultants had relationships with community staff, the consultants would not be able to hold the communities accountable. I can only wonder how parents have been able to hold their children accountable for millennia if this belief were true. That one belief is now preventing us from engaging in necessary organizational redesign. You see how formal leaders' beliefs that have unconsciously formed into paradigms have a huge impact on an organization and can either promote or prevent growth. They can cause paradigm paralysis, the inability to see beyond your own beliefs.

I tried to think of all of the responsibilities of a leader in a care community. Then I took each of those areas of responsibility and identified the shift in thinking that must occur to become a person-centered leader. I next invited a group of amazing person-centered administrators to join me in identifying the accompanying behavior shifts that must occur to create a context for a truly caring community. Over the next several pages, I offer you the fruits of our labor: the Person-Centered Leader Quick Reference Matrix, a tool to help you shift your beliefs and, hopefully, your behaviors. By changing your behavior, you will begin to change the context of your community, which is what I will address more fully in the next chapter. Enjoy!

PERSON-CENTERED LEADER QUICK REFERENCE MATRIX

AREA OF RESPONSIBILITY	THINKING SHIFTS	BEHAVIOR SHIFTS
RELATIONSHIP BUILDING	Think community instead of institution. In a human community, people are well known to each other. These relationships are the key to my success.	Practice engagement; make decisions by principles not emotions; adopt compassion & curiosity; listen first; grow trust by becoming vulnerable; over-communicate honestly and openly; set a standard for conduct; give people the tools to walk beside you
INTERNAL RELATIONSHIPS		
Relationships with Residents	1. One of the most important roles I play as a leader is as the residents' advocate. 2. Residents have a right to direct their own lives, to be well known in the community, and to be a partner in their own care by participating in decisions that affect their lives. They do not have to bend to the will of the organization. 3. Residents have a right to live a life of purpose, not just one spent waiting to die. 4. Rounds are a vehicle for relationship building, as well as a way to identify opportunities for improvement. 5. Complaints are good! In a human community, when they feel safe and when they believe it will make a difference, people complain.	1. Help the residents become deeply known in the community. 2. Question your motives and your practices to ensure that all you do is based on what is best for each resident at that time. Residents rule; they make the decisions about their own lives. Your role is to protect, sustain, and nurture the residents, not control them. 3. Hold daily community meetings where the residents' voices are heard. 4. Rounds are more than walking the halls. Smile, look relaxed. While making rounds, answer call lights, and, if you can, help the resident. Make a point of asking the residents questions that will help them become more well known to you. 5. All complaints, concerns, and compliments should be met with gratitude and appreciation for the gift they truly are. By sharing a complaint or concern, a resident is showing that he trusts you and believes that you will address the problem. Of course, you do not want the same complaint to be made again and again. That means you are not growing.

Relationships with Families	1. Families are our care partners, not our antagonists. The "good" family is one who is present and attentive as well as questions and challenges us to be the best we can be for their loved one. The care partner relationship with the family must be clarified and defined prior to or upon admission. 2. Families need a voice in the community, other than through the complaint/concern process.	1. Give your staff a different view of the families who visit often and complain frequently. Frame them as "good" families who are attentive and caring of their loved ones. Complaints are really gifts that need to be appreciated. They raise our awareness of things that need improvement so that we can elevate the art of caregiving. Try to discover the ways that families want to continue to participate in giving care to their loved ones, so that they can continue to play an important role in their care. Offer them other ways they can contribute besides complaining. When they do share a concern, engage them in being part of the solution. 2. Take charge of the family council process and help families understand that the true purpose of the council is to bring families into the decision making, planning, goal setting, and process improvement of the community.
Relationships with Staff	1. Organizational climate affects everyone, especially the residents. I am responsible for the climate in my community. 2. I am the resource bearer, barrier buster, customer advocate, results guardian, facilitator, educator, guide, and coach, not the boss. I grow people. To do that, I have to grow myself first. 3. Control is a myth. The only person I can control is myself. 4. I must make every effort to know my staff well and show them I care about them.	1. As a leadership team, we need to examine everything we are doing and saying, as well as all of our policies. Put them to the test using The Eden Alternative® Golden Rule: "As management does unto staff, so shall staff do unto the Elders." 2. Lose the idea that you are "in charge," and adopt the idea that you grow people. Create a climate where each person can be the best he or she can be for the world. 3. You no longer have the answers, only the questions. 4. Knowing your staff requires more than just walking up and down the hallways every day. It requires a genuine interest and effort in knowing them as human beings with families, interests, and feelings, just like you.

AREA OF RESPONSIBILITY	THINKING SHIFTS	BEHAVIOR SHIFTS
Relationships with Volunteers	Volunteers are an important and vital part of our community. They serve us in many ways. Through proper planning, engagement, training, support, and recognition, we can enjoy the benefits of many different volunteers. As a leader of my community, I must initiate and facilitate that kind of planning and support.	In the institutional culture, we believed that volunteers just appear at our door, and we should be thankful for them. In a person-centered culture, creating and sustaining a robust, vigorous, and diverse volunteer force is a function of your leadership.
EXTERNAL RELATIONSHIPS		
Relationships with Consultants	Consultants are a resource and source of expertise for our communities, not a punitive oversight team. They are not in our community to rescue; they are here to educate and grow capacity in me and my staff. They are part of our team.	Include your consultants in the teams and improvement process within your community. Be willing to hold the consultants to the same code of conduct to which you hold yourselves and your staff. At the same time, help staff build strong relationships with their consultants so that they see them for the resource they are, not another fault-finder or enabler.
Relationships with Medical Director/ Physicians	The medical director and other physicians are our care partners and an important resource in improving the well-being of our residents. They are not God, nor the boss of the residents. They are, however, important community members who bring great value to assist in protecting, nurturing, and sustaining our residents.	Physicians must understand that although they play an important role, the resident is in charge of her own life. Physicians need to be educated on the standards of conduct for the community and should understand our person-centered philosophy (which is embodied in statute F155: Residents have the right to refuse medical treatment).
Relationships with Home Office Staff	The people who work at the home office are my guides, resource bearers, mentors, barrier busters, and support. They are not fault-finders, finger-pointers, or blame-shifters. I can go to them for knowledge, training, support, and problem solving. I can support their mission in many ways, including participating in meetings and education, offering support to my sister communities, and serving on task forces, such as the one that developed this guide. Together we are indomitable. I am proud to be a part of an organization that is leading the way in innovative models of care.	Recognize and appreciate the resources and support of the home office team. Build strong relationships with them. Communicate respectfully with them, acknowledge their contributions to your own success, and exercise patience with them, understanding that they serve several communities. Encourage your staff to do the same. Be supportive of, and at times participate in, new initiatives, challenges, new opportunities. A positive, "can do" attitude will endear you to the (just as) hard-working people at the home office.

Relationships with Larger Community	We are an important and vital part of our larger community. We have many resources, including the richness of our elders, that we can share. There are many resources available in the larger community that we can enjoy. It is my responsibility to engage and connect our community with the larger community, so that we may all enjoy these reciprocal relationships.	Reach out across the illusionary divide and re-create connections with the larger community.
Relationships with Governmental Agencies	I want to be influencing policies, rules, and regulations that will affect my community. Strong relationships with local, state, and federal governmental agencies will help me do that.	Attend advisory meetings with your state regulatory agency. Meet your Ombudsman, and build a strong relationship with her. She is an important resource for you and your residents.
ACTIVITIES	Providing meaningful activities, both planned and spontaneous, requires everyone's participation, not just the activity department. We are all responsible for meeting the social, recreational, emotional, and spiritual needs of our residents.	Inspire a new view that we are all responsible for meeting the needs of the human spirit, then begin the process of cross-training and engaging all staff in the delivery of meaningful activities, both planned and spontaneous. Managers conduct at least one activity per month with residents.
ADMISSIONS	1. Moving into a new community is a large life event that can impact every domain of well-being. 2. Hands-on staff must be involved in the inquiry and admission process, so that they "know" the elder before she arrives. The shift in thinking must extend to hands-on staff who have a role in welcoming and comforting the elder in her new home. Trust must be shifted from the admissions director to the care partners. 3. Simple pleasures and daily routines bring meaning into our lives. We must discover the simple pleasures and daily routines of new residents, and help them maintain them in their lives. 4. For transitional care residents: Although this is not their home, while they are with us, they will enjoy the comforts of home. Knowing them well is the path to providing those comforts. 5. Assessments of new residents should include strengths, not just deficits.	1. Make sure that moving into a community is as gentle, nurturing, welcoming, reassuring, and hopeful as possible for the resident. Have each neighborhood design its own welcome ritual. 2. Huddle on the neighborhood to present the information about a new resident. Create strong relationships between the hospital liaisons and hands-on staff. Discuss ways to shift trust from the admissions person to the hands-on staff. 3. Discover each resident's simple pleasures. Have the hands-on teams decide how to support and maintain those pleasure. Include simple pleasures on the care plans. 4. Find out as much as possible about things that will bring a new resident comfort. Communicate those things to the hands-on staff, and make sure those items are in place when the new resident arrives. 5. Communicate a new view of aging as developmental aging. Engage all of your staff in efforts to identify and nurture the growth of each of your residents.

AREA OF RESPONSIBILITY	THINKING SHIFTS	BEHAVIOR SHIFTS
BUSINESS DEVELOPMENT	We are entrepreneurs, enjoying the risks and rewards of our community. We must care for the business as if it is our own.	Constantly imagine new ways to grow your business. Communicate the larger business environment picture to all of your stakeholders.
BUSINESS OFFICE	1. To create a caring and sustainable community, we must all become good fiscal stewards of the community's assets. My role is not only monitoring those assets, but also teaching others how to become good stewards. The NHA and BOM are the not the only ones who can care for the financial resources of the community. I will never say "We can't afford it" or "We don't have the budget for it." Instead, I will educate people about the budget, and ask them how we can make something happen if it is important to us. 2. Cross-training other staff in noncritical components of the business office will provide the opportunity for the BOM to come out of her office and participate in the life of the community.	1. Educate everyone on budgets, payor sources, and per patient days. Instead of, "We don't have the budget for it," try saying, "If that is something that you believe is important for our residents or our community, let's talk about how we can make that happen." You are then challenging them to find a way. Through that process, a lot of education can occur. It can also make room for creativity, passion, and commitment. NHAs still need to take responsibility and daily stay on top of all of the business office functions. 2. Cross-train other staff in nonessential functions in the business office. That way, the BOM can come out and enjoy other aspects of life in the community.
CARE CONFERENCES	Care conferences are for capturing the resident's story, goals, wishes, strengths, well-being needs, and simple pleasures.	Include the resident and those closest to her, her family, and her hands-on care partners, in the care conference. Consider rethinking where they are held. If possible, go to the resident's room, where she can be comfortable and the assessment team can evaluate her in her environment. As a leader, attend as many care conferences as you can. Include in the care plan the resident's wishes, goals, strengths, well-being needs, and simple pleasures. Ask the hands-on care partners who attend the conference to hold a huddle with the rest of their team to share the results of the care conference, so that everyone knows the plan of care.

CARE COORDINATION	Our responsibility to our residents begins before they arrive and does not stop when they are discharged to another level of care or to home. We must put systems into place to ensure that the transitions between environments protects and serves our residents.	Have in place people and systems that will ensure smooth transitions. Case managers must provide important communication and follow up that protects the residents and ensures that care continues prior to a resident's arrival and even after he or she has left your community. Building strong relationships with other care providers in the continuum of care will help ensure good communication and smooth transitions.
CENSUS MANAGEMENT	Maximizing the resources of the community through good census management will protect and sustain the community. Everyone in my organization should have knowledge about Medicare and Medicaid and why it is important to manage the census in today's world.	Educate your staff about the realities of our reimbursement systems, a chronically underfunded system, and the narrow margins that threaten our very existence. This education must be accompanied by the communication of a strong vision of how we can continue as a care community if we work together to meet our challenges. The entire leadership team must discuss census management daily in the morning meeting. And the community, including the hands-on care partners, should be engaged in discussions about managing any necessary transfers with the least impact to residents.
CLINICAL REIMBURSEMENT	1. We go where the resident takes us, not one step less or one step further. It is our obligation to ensure each resident is provided all services that are needed and that we are paid for the services we provide. 2. Old thinking perceives documentation as a burden to meet regulatory requirements. New thinking sees documentation as capturing the elder's story to raise the art of caregiving to its highest level.	1. Ensure that each person receives the services she needs to reach her maximum potential. We do not over-treat or under-treat. As a leader, you must ensure that optimal treatment is being received by each resident. Attend and be engaged in your daily PPS meeting. 2. Communicate to all staff that residents' stories must be documented and that those stories help us raise the art of caregiving to its highest level. It is not only our means of reimbursement, but our means of communicating the needs and desires of the residents across all disciplines and all shifts. Educate staff to ensure all documentation supports the services delivered. Do not bill for services that are not supported by proper documentation.

AREA OF RESPONSIBILITY	THINKING SHIFTS	BEHAVIOR SHIFTS
CORPORATE COMPLIANCE	Ensuring that all of our actions and the actions of our staff are ethically and legally sound protects our community and its residents. Integrity of the highest order in everything we do is imperative.	*"Do what is right, proper, and good."* Educate the community that there are no secrets and that each of us, no matter our title, will be held accountable to higher standards of conduct. We do not lie, cheat, steal, falsify, or cover up mistakes. As a leader, you are also responsible for ensuring that all of our billing is accurate and appropriate. We do not bill for services that we have not performed nor have the proper documentation for. You will ensure that the resident trust account is balanced and accurate. You must also ensure that resident health information is protected and that staff maintain the confidentiality of all resident issues according to the HIPPA regulations.
DIETARY SERVICES	1. Food is not just a cost center. It is one of the last great pleasures in a human life. The mechanical, industrialized approach to food is harming our residents. Elders deserve to eat the foods that they enjoy, when and where they want to enjoy them. 2. Meal time provides our residents with much more than nutrition and hydration. It provides our residents with "convivium," the opportunity to share "good food with good friends." This is an opportunity to create and deepen meaning. 3. Elders deserve "refrigerator rights." 4. Meal service is one of the most important times in our residents' lives. Formal leaders need to be present, engaged, involved, and in service at every meal.	1. Replace institutional practices with resident involvement in the planning, preparation, design, and enjoyment of their own dining experience. Liberalize diet orders and dining committees, and expand choice and dining hours. 2. Dining is not just a task completed on a set schedule three times a day per regulations. Meal times need to be a time of convivium, when people in our communities have a sense they are "nourishing their spirit" and enhancing relationships, as well as feeding their bodies. 3. Having food, not just any food, but the food your residents and staff enjoy available 24 hours a day is vital to creating a caring community. Depending on your community, not only its unique physical design, but the uniqueness of your residents, this opportunity may take shape in many different forms. 4. Set the standard of conduct for all managers around meal service. Our management teams create a schedule that puts at least one manager in each dining room for each meal.

EMERGENCY PREPAREDNESS	Having a plan and training everyone to that plan creates a calmness that comes from confidence during a real disaster that ensures the well-being of everyone in the community.	This is an ethical responsibility that must not be taken lightly. You must establish a plan for order and crisis leadership and then educate everyone to that plan.
EQUIPMENT/ SUPPLY MANAGEMENT	I am a resource bearer and a protector of the community's resources. I must share my expertise, knowledge, and information with everyone, so that everyone is invested in: 1. Making sure our residents have the supplies and equipment they need when they need it. 2. Ensuring that all equipment is functioning properly. 3. Making sure we are all good stewards of our resources, so that we are not paying for things we do not need or keeping equipment that does not work, cannot be repaired, or is no longer needed. Nor are we wasting resources or energy in managing equipment and supplies. Scarcity mentality does not produce cost-saving behaviors; it only produces hoarding and stinginess. Education about budgets and supply resources, a well-organized and well-stocked central supply, and ensuring that the hands-on staff have what they need to care for the residents will ensure efficiency, effectiveness, and cost-containment.	You are a resource bearer. Make sure everyone has what they need to care for the residents. Hold learning circles with hands-on staff to communicate that you want them to have what they need, and that you want them to deliver the very best care. Find out their challenges regarding equipment and supplies. Do not speak or act in terms of scarcity. Educate and engage everyone in becoming good stewards of resources.
ETHICS	I must engage the community in struggling to find the right thing to do each day.	In a human community, we join together with guiding principles and discuss how to apply these principles to the decisions at hand. As wisdom is not found in one person's head, the community engages in dialog around what can often be very challenging issues in our world of long-term care. Utilize the Principles for Ethical Decision Making. Create and attend a monthly Code of Ethics committee.

AREA OF RESPONSIBILITY	THINKING SHIFTS	BEHAVIOR SHIFTS
FINANCIAL MANAGEMENT/ INTERNAL CONTROLS	I must share the accountability for our financial well-being with the other stakeholders in the community. It will take all of us to make the best financial decisions for our community.	Educate and engage stakeholders in the community about budgets. Monitor your budget and your financial outcomes weekly and monthly. The NHA is accountable for ensuring all internal control compliance over financial reporting for your community. It is important that she ensure the accuracy of information through the monitoring of all financial systems.
FRONT DESK	1. First impressions are lasting. 2. Receptionists have important information to share. 3. Overhead paging is an archaic practice and should be discontinued, except in the event of an emergency.	1. Recognize the importance of first impressions and know that the person who you place into that role will set the tone of the experience for each person who enters your community. 2. Include the receptionist in important information, and gather information from her. 3. Create a policy that dictates the elimination of overhead paging.
HOUSEKEEPING	1. It is everyone's job to ensure our community is clean and safe for all of us. 2. Housekeepers are an important part of the care team and have important information that can help us raise the art of care partnering. Residents often speak to housekeepers more than any other employee.	1. Communicate and model that anything that is not required by license or certification can be done by anyone. Communicate clearly that it is everyone's job to make sure that the community is kept clean and safe. 2. Consistently assign housekeepers to every neighborhood. Have them participate in neighborhood and community meetings. Include them in huddles after an incident. They have valuable information. Consult residents and housekeepers for feedback about environmental changes and systems. Communicate that the housekeepers' eyes and voices are much needed. Communicate to the housekeepers that they have an equal voice in learning circles and problem solving.

HUMAN RESOURCES	*"As management does unto staff, so shall staff do unto the elders."*
1. We are a business for people, by people. Human resources are our greatest assets.	1. Put everything you and your management team do to the test of this rule.
2. Potential new community members should be interviewed by the residents, families, and staff.	2. Involve residents, staff, and, if possible, families in the interview process.
3. We must create a just culture and not rely upon the punitive culture. Accountability is about growth, not punishment.	3. Redefine accountability as growth, not punishment. Do not punish people for making mistakes, only for reckless behavior. Use the Accountability Survey to help in making decisions regarding employee accountability.
4. My staff is smart. They want to do a good job. They can make good decisions when the empowerment conditions are met.	4. Empowerment is a function of leadership. It requires the leaders' ongoing participation not as the decision makers, but as the guides who bring knowledge, training and skills, information, resources, and a supportive environment to the teams. These are the empowerment conditions that must be met in order to effectively move decision-making authority.
5. My staff is just like me. They motivate themselves when the intrinsic motivators are present.	5. Create an environment, climate, and culture where people are motivated to be the best they can be because the three intrinsic motivators are present: autonomy, mastery, and meaning.
INFORMATION/ DATA MANAGE- MENT	1. Make data and information actionable. As a person-centered leader, data will become a large part of your decision-making process. Tracking and trending important information can give you early warning signs of problems that may occur.
1. I rely on good information and measurable outcomes to ensure the well-being of the residents, their families, the staff, and the community. Empirical data is an important tool in creating a caring community.	2. Become transparent. While you "own" the data (making sure they are accurate), you also "share" them with all stakeholders, engaging them in process improvement.
2. I utilize data throughout the community, sharing outcome data and engaging all stakeholders in process improvement.	3. We use many different types of indicators to inform our work and progress, but our greatest measure of success is the well-being and satisfaction of our residents, their families, and our employees.
3. We measure the well-being and satisfaction of our stakeholders as our greatest outcome.	

AREA OF RESPONSIBILITY	THINKING SHIFTS	BEHAVIOR SHIFTS
LAUNDRY	1. Our residents' personal clothing and possessions are an important part of their identity. They should be treated with the utmost respect. 2. Residents and families who choose to do so should have access to personal laundry equipment to care for their own clothes.	1. Pay more attention to how we are treating the personal possessions and clothing of our residents. Work with your staff to develop effective systems. Support staff and residents in having learning circles and/or laundry committees to come up with solutions for personal laundry. Purchase a labeling machine and make sure staff have the supplies and training to use it. 2. Find a way to install personal laundry machines in your community. Make sure that you know the laundry regulations better than the surveyors.
LOCAL/STATE/ NATIONAL PRESENCE	1. We are part of a larger community that influences the well-being of our community. My leadership extends beyond the walls of this community, so that the voices of my elders, staff, and families can be heard. 2. Participation in and demonstration of the quality of life we provide our residents is more than a star on our chests. Participation helps us in our continual improvement, acknowledges the hard work of our staff, and shows the world that it can be different.	1. You act as the voice of your community, participating on a local, state, and national level as its spokesperson. Participate in the political process and involve all of your stakeholders. 2. Participate in awards programs that showcase the work that you do, as well as drive your own process improvement. Know the five-star program and how you can improve or maintain your star level.
MAINTENANCE	1. Our residents deserve to have a well-maintained, comfortable, and safe home environment. 2. Maintenance people have many talents that can benefit our community.	1. Daily monitor the physical environment for comfort, safety, and appearance. Leaders need a base of knowledge to know when things are not right. They communicate to everyone that each person needs to be looking out for things that need repair or attention. Person-centered leaders are proactive in their approach to maintenance. They hire for the kind of skills their building requires. They know the scope of practice of their maintenance person and understand what kinds of things will require an outside contractor. 2. Free up time for the maintenance person to share those talents in many different ways, including creating "home" in the physical environment, participating in activity programming, and educating staff.

MARKETING	1. Everyone in our community is a marketing person and a storyteller. 2. The best marketing we can do is building relationships internally and externally.	1. Have hands-on staff and/or residents give tours and provide testimony to families about why they should bring their loved one to your community. Capture and collect those positive stories and share them in many different ways: verbally in presentations to community groups or to referral sources, on your webpage, in your newsletter, and everywhere you and your staff go. 2. You change people's perceptions about long-term care, especially your community, through the development of strong relationships with your internal and external stakeholders. This is the best marketing you can do.
MEDICAL RECORDS	1. Proper documentation tells the residents' stories and elevates the art of care partnering. 2. Proper documentation protects our community and releases us from fear-based decisions and actions.	1. Educate staff on the most important reason we must be diligent in the pursuit of documentation: to tell the story of each resident so that we can elevate the art of care partnering. A core value of person-centered care is to know each person. In this model, the medical record becomes the story that we share with all care partners to help each resident become well known. 2. When we are comfortable that we are truly telling the story of our residents in their medical records, that those records are complete and accurate, and that they are protected for privacy and confidentiality, we can release the fear of deficiencies, fines, lawsuits, and the refunding of Medicare or Medicaid resources. Released from that fear, we can make the best decisions based on our ethical principles.
MEETINGS	Meetings are an important means of communicating in a human community. They must have clarity of purpose, include all stakeholders' voices, be organized, have ground rules, result in action plans, and be evaluated for improvement.	Set the context for meaningful, productive meetings. Learn good meeting facilitation skills and use them.

AREA OF RESPONSIBILITY	THINKING SHIFTS	BEHAVIOR SHIFTS
NURSING	1. Medical treatment is a servant of genuine human caring, never its master. Nursing is to support residents' lives not to be the center of their lives. 2. Residents have the right to autonomy over their daily lives, including the right to refuse treatment and the right to risk in the pursuit of happiness. We work around residents' lives and do not expect them to work around our schedules.	1. Educate everyone on genuine human caring and how sometimes nursing care is within the scope of that practice, and sometimes outside the scope. When we use medical treatment to master the resident, it is harmful not caring. 2. Be diligent in advocating for your residents' rights while doing everything you can to protect our community.
PERSONAL LEADERSHIP DEVELOPMENT	An organization rises to the level of its formal leadership. I must grow myself first, and then grow others to be leaders.	Understand that your growth is vital to the success of your community. The leadership journey is a lifelong pursuit in search of honing your skills as a leader, so that your community can continue its path of growth. Grow yourself first, then reach out and grow leadership in others.
PHARMACY	1. This community will never resort to the use of drugs for staff convenience. We must make sure the clinical team is trained on nonpharmacological interventions and has access to tools to use before they use a drug. There must be an ongoing, united effort to reduce the use of pharmaceuticals that are not serving our residents. 2. Drugs can ease suffering, but they can also kill. The use of antipsychotics in people living with dementia is mostly contraindicated and can cause premature death.	1. The effort to reduce the use of pharmaceuticals in a person-centered community is a united effort between the leadership of the community, the physicians, the pharmacy and pharmacy consultants, and the hands-on staff. 2. Change the paradigm and the language of "behaviors" to put the onus on us, not the residents. When a resident exhibits a "behavior" that we do not like or find inappropriate, that resident is really expressing an "unmet need." Now it is up to us, the care partners, to try to figure out what need is not being met. I doubt it is a need for another pill. Knowing the resident well will help staff in identifying what need is not being met.

PHYSICAL PLANT	1. This is our residents' home. Home is an important part of our identity and, therefore, our well-being. 2. This is where we work, and people deserve a nice place to work.	1. Engage the community, residents, and staff in making the best use of the spaces you have available. Know your residents well, and then create a home that reflects those residents. 2. Listen to your staff and remove any barriers in the physical plant that may be contributing to added stress or increased work for the care partners. Have a comfortable, attractive space for staff to take their breaks. Give the staff some funds and let them paint, furnish, and decorate the space the way they would like.
POLICIES & PROCEDURES	1. Institutions use policies and procedures in an attempt to control the uncontrollable. Communities use best practices, principles, and values to create a stable, effective, efficient, and caring environment. 2. Show me a man-made rule, and I'll show you an exception. 3. Policies and procedures should represent best practices. Best practices change as we grow and learn more. We need to review our policies and procedures regularly to ensure they are kept current with our practices.	1. Encourage your staff to challenge the current processes, continually seeking a better way. If the current policy and procedure is not serving your residents, your staff, or the organization, then consider changing it. If it is a policy and procedure developed at your home office, then advocate for changing it. 2. Make decisions on principles rather than rules. 3. Review policies frequently to ensure they represent the current best practices.
QUALITY ASSURANCE/ PROCESS IMPROVEMENT (QAPI)	1. Quality assurance and process improvement (QAPI) is everyone's job, not just the leadership team's. 2. Process improvement does not wait for the monthly meeting. It is a daily practice.	1. Use data and process improvement throughout your community, engaging everyone in this continuous effort of improvement. Learning and teaching everyone the tools of process improvement are critical to your role as the leader of a caring community. 2. Person-centered leaders do not use QAPI because it is required by regulation. They use it because they know it is the path to excellence and to improving the lives of the people who live and work in their communities. They not only review clinical outcomes, but are also continually looking, sharing, reviewing, analyzing, and doing root-cause analysis and action planning around all of their outcome data. It does not wait for the monthly meeting. It is a part of the daily lives of all care partners.

AREA OF RESPONSIBILITY	THINKING SHIFTS	BEHAVIOR SHIFTS
RISK MANAGEMENT/ SAFETY/OSHA	1. Fear-based thinking and behaviors put our community at more risk than principle-based thinking and behaviors. The best risk management I can do is in building strong relationships. 2. Surplus safety is just as dangerous as too little safety. We strive for optimal safety. 3. We are proactive in managing risk. And when an accident happens, we conduct root-cause analysis, problem-solving, and action planning to try to prevent it from happening again.	1. The best risk management you can do is building strong relationships with all stakeholders in your community and doing what is right every time. Act with integrity and transparency because you have nothing to hide. 2. Surplus safety only sees one side of risk—the down side. It tells us that all risk is bad and that there will be negative consequences if we engage in risk. But there is another side of risk—the upside. This is the advantage we receive when we risk in the pursuit of happiness. If we try to remove all risk, we also remove the upside of risk, which deals a crushing blow to the human spirit, putting residents at even more risk. 3. Too much safety is harmful, that is true. But so is too little safety. What we need in a caring community is optimal safety.
SOCIAL SERVICES	1. The well-being of the human spirit is just as important as the well-being of the human body. 2. "Behaviors" are expressions of unmet needs, not problems. The onus is on the care partners to figure out what need is not being met and to try to meet it, not on the resident to "behave."	1. Acknowledge the value and importance of the social workers and the services they provide, and elevate their importance in your community as equal to care of the body. 2. "Behaviors" are actually expressions of an unmet need. We now have to discover what need is being unmet. In a person-centered world, we know each resident and their families well. This helps us in knowing what might alleviate an unmet need. We have the consistent care partners for our residents so that they can develop deeper relationships.

STAFF DEVELOPMENT	1. The more I invest in the growth of my staff, the stronger our community will be. 2. I must manage conflict in my community so that it does not bleed over onto the residents.	1. Develop a robust and creative staff development program that engages all staff in the learning process. 2. In a true person-centered world where every person is taught the skills of conflict resolution, where conflict mediators are available, and where there is a new standard of conduct, conflict becomes a positive rather than destructive force. It becomes the way we understand each other. It becomes the way we find the most creative solutions because we are not afraid to challenge processes and systems. And we can do that because we do it respectfully.
SURVEY MANAGEMENT	1. Survey outcomes are no longer my greatest measure of success. 2. We are not guilty of anything other than doing our best every day. 3. Surveyors are part of my quality improvement team, not the enemy.	1. Survey outcomes are just one measure of success. Your focus is on providing the best care you can using the best practices you have, and you do that every day, not just when you are in your survey window. 2. Impress on your staff that this is just another day. Whether the surveyors are in the building or not, you will do the same thing you do every day. You are not guilty of anything other than doing your best every day. 3. The state surveyors are not your enemy. They are part of your process improvement team. Shifting this paradigm takes the pressure off you and your staff.
TEAM DEVELOPMENT	1. Wisdom is not found in one person's head. I cannot do this alone. 2. The answers to all of our problems are within this community to discover.	1. Believe in the power of teams. Teams are essential to your success and the success of your community in the future. We can no longer work in a century-old model to deliver care in the new world. The first and most critical team that must be developed is your leadership team. 2. Person-centered leaders are leading the way, not sitting back and waiting for circumstances to determine their future and the future of their community. They are driving the future. And because they have strong trusting teams, their organizations also have the flexibility to respond very quickly to change in the external environment.

AREA OF RESPONSIBILITY	THINKING SHIFTS	BEHAVIOR SHIFTS
THERAPY	1. Human growth must never be separated from human life. 2. Therapists are an important part of our care partner team.	1. Therapy services can support a full and abundant life. These services should be available to everyone, despite diagnosis or payor source. This will require you to develop strong restorative nursing services to back up the therapy team. Get creative and screen and plan for each resident who will benefit from these services. This does not mean you force people into services or that you overtreat. You always "go where the resident takes us; not one step less or further." 2. The therapists are engaged and involved as a vital part of the care partner team. They attend daily PPS meetings with the IDT. They are aware of and participate in more than just their department. It is your job as a person-centered leader to include them in as many things as possible and make sure they are trained in a person-centered philosophy. They must understand that they will bend to the daily schedules of our residents, not the other way around.
WELL-BEING	The ultimate measure of success for your community is the well-being of all.	The Seven Domains of Well-Being Identity Connectedness Security Autonomy Meaning Growth Joy The Eden Alternative Domains of Well-Being™ frame a conversation that can be used throughout the organization. The more they become a focal point in growth plans (care plans and performance evaluations), care partner team meetings, education, decision making, and problem solving, the more likely it is that everyone on the team will experience well-being.

CHAPTER 7

Solving the Problem

Changing the Context

Organizational Redesign

Architecture does not create extraordinary organizations by collecting extraordinary people. It does so by enabling very ordinary people to perform in extraordinary ways.

—John Kay, economist

Person-centered leaders cannot stop at changing beliefs. Leadership Truth #2 teaches us about the power of context in shaping human behavior. Just as I was able to solve the problem with my mother by changing the context of our relationship, so, too, can formal leaders change the context of their care communities. In the lessons for this chapter, I discuss some of the more important ways to change the context of care communities to create sustainable person-centered care.

The biggest culprit in shaping the behavior of people working in care communities is the very organizational design of all our care communities. The institutional model taught us to organize our work into departmental silos, each managed by a department manager in a top-down hierarchy designed to ensure the timely and efficient execution of a series of tasks and procedures. Managers hire and train staff and then monitor them to ensure they are doing their jobs. The work in a care community is divided into small chunks with a robust delineation between job positions. All of the accountabilities in the organization go up the departmental silos through an active chain of command. Those closest to the elders hold very little, if any, decision-making authority.

I can enter almost any of the nearly 16,000 skilled nursing facilities in the United States, as well as in many other countries that have followed this same type of organizational design, and find many of the same staff behaviors. And this is despite the fact that the people working in these communities are from completely different cultures.

Organizational architectures are purposeful interventions, designed to shape human behavior. And none has done a better job of shaping human behavior than the one we have adopted in our care communities. I most likely have not visited your care community, but I can tell you what happens there on a daily basis. I can tell you what kinds of behaviors exist among your staff. If you have followed the typical organizational design of the institutional model, I would bet that you have ongoing, unmitigated conflict between departments, shifts, and management staff and hands-on staff. You most likely have some misunderstandings and resentments between nurses and CNAs. I can tell you that your staff is most likely task driven and worry that they might do more work than the other shifts or departments or even their peers. I am going to bet there is a plethora of gossip, judgment, and blame happening daily. I am also going to guess that most employees will tell you they do not have enough staff and are feeling overwhelmed. Some of you may have even tried to mitigate this problem by adding positions or breaking down the already limited jobs into even smaller, more specialized jobs (e.g., bath aides, feeding assistants). Do you have the same problems happening over and over, and, no matter what you try, they never get solved? Is there resistance to change in your community? Does the vast majority of your turnover happen in the first 6 months of employment? Do you have employees who call off their shifts repeatedly? Does this occur mostly on weekends? I am going to guess that you have a handful of department managers who work long hours, tirelessly trying to support those hands-on employees who will not be held accountable.

How did I do? The fact that you have chosen this book tells me that some of these problems have most likely been alleviated through your leadership. But why does almost every nursing home have these same behaviors and problems? It is because they have all used the same organizational design and leadership style. The irony of that statement is that there is no regulation that tells us how to organize our work. There is no law about how to lead. The regulations tell us what, not how. The law tells you not to discriminate in your leadership practices; that is all.

The other irony is that all of these care communities have been following a century-old management theory that has been abandoned by most other industries, some of them more than 50 years ago. In the early 1900s, many management theorists attempted to better understand how businesses could become more efficient through the use of scientific methods. They conducted time studies in manufacturing plants. They promoted the idea of the division of labor into specialty tasks. They believed that managers should train their workers to perform these tasks and then monitor them closely to ensure that they were doing their tasks in the most scientifically proven efficient manner.

One of the most influential of these theorists was Frederick Taylor, an engineer who published *The Principles of Scientific Management* in 1911. His management theory espoused one right way to do a task based on the science. Managers were responsible for training staff in that right way and monitoring them to ensure compliance. He maintained that workers should be matched to specialized tasks that fit their abilities. He also believed that workers who were more productive should be rewarded more, as their only motivation was money. One practice that "Taylorism" also promoted was bringing together management and staff, which has led to more modern management practices. Prior to his theory, managers rarely had contact with workers (Sandrone, 1997).

In the early part of the 20th century, most manufacturers adopted Taylor's management theory. But by the end of the century, most had deserted the practice. Taylorism did make significant contributions to improving productivity and working conditions for employees, but it was fraught with problems. Among these, the most injurious was "destroying the soul of work, dehumanizing factories, and making men into automatons" (Sandrone, 1997).

Prior to factories and scientific management, work was performed by craftsmen and their apprentices. These craftsmen acted as masters over their work. They had the ability to design and plan their work, their time, and their tasks. They were able to evaluate the quality of their work and guide process improvements. Since Deming and the process improvement movement that began in Japan, many manufacturers have moved away from Taylorism as well as the division of labor and the top-down hierarchy that came with it. They have discovered that Taylorism stripped the meaning out of their employees' work. It removed them from having any say in how that work was performed or any input into the evaluation of that work. In dehumanizing the workers, it actually created a context in which people were demotivated.

And, yet, here we are in our care communities clinging to an outdated management theory and organizational design that manufacturers have proven does not work. When faced with the poor outcomes of this way of organizing our work, we try to break down the tasks even further. We adopt an even more directing, micromanaging, and controlling management style. We are in the business of care, yet we are dehumanizing and demotivating our care force. At the same time, we are running our department managers ragged, expecting them to be the only accountable ones.

It is time for us to admit that the way we have been organizing our work is contrary to our mission of creating a care community where everyone can experience well-being. It is the big culprit in many of our problems. It has created a context for human behavior that none of us like. And there is nothing stopping us from changing it.

Let us take a look at how we organize ourselves at home. At home, we do not have a dietary department or a housekeeping department. At home, we do not organize our work in departments. At home, we work as teams. Our accountabilities do not go up some department silo to a department manager. At home, we are accountable to each other. We care about each other. We help each other. At home, we are all cross-trained. We can do each other's jobs.

Whereas Taylorism and scientific management promoted the specialization of labor, person-centered care understands that our success lies in our ability to be flexible. Cross-training creates flexibility. There is no possible way to meet the individual needs and desires of 100 elders without that kind of flexibility.

Dr. Bill Thomas says, "Make the job as big as their hearts" (personal communication, 2003). In his Green House® model, the CNAs are cross-trained in cooking, housekeeping, laundry, and activities. They are able to meet the elders' needs at the point of service. True, this is possible because of the physical transformation into small houses equipped with a kitchen and laundry. The question, however, is how can we expand the role of our care partners, given the limitations of our physical environment? Can we put a pantry kitchen or serving kitchen on our neighborhoods? Can we put personal laundry machines on each neighborhood? Can we cross-train our CNAs and housekeepers? Can we train everyone as a CNA? That does not mean everyone works as a CNA, but that they are available if an elder needs assistance. Can we train everyone in activities and have them bring their passions to share with the elders? Can we cross-train our managers? Do not use your traditional physical plant as an excuse for not cross-training.

The other factor that impedes flexibility is hierarchy. If a CNA has to stop what she is doing to ask permission to meet the needs of an elder, the elder's needs will not be met. The hierarchy is too unwieldy, cumbersome, and time-consuming. So, not only do we need cross-training, we need empowerment. And the crowning touch to this new way of organizing your work is to develop high-functioning, self-managed, and cross-functional teams. I wrote in Lesson 10 about our own efforts at Vivage to do this through the Neighborhood Guide Training we developed. We have since licensed that curriculum to The Eden Alternative, so it is available to everyone through their educators.

SHIFTING ACCOUNTABILITY

As you begin to create empowered teams, you begin to shift the accountability out of your departmental silos and into the teams. This is critical. Under the institutional system, only a few people are accountable because they hold all of the authority. As you begin to move decision-making authority into the neighborhood teams, do not forget that accountability comes with that authority. One way to begin that process is by having the team create their own Code of Ethics, rather than handing one to them. We have plenty of hierarchical rules. We do not need more of those. What we need for a team to be high functioning is peer accountability, which is much more powerful than any formal rules we might devise. It is much faster, more effective, and highly motivational. The United States military does a remarkable job in creating peer accountability among young men and women from all parts of the country, various cultures, and beliefs. This sense of belonging is so powerful that these young people will risk their lives for each other. You may not be able to attain that level of accountability, but you can create a context in which the anxiety of not meeting the expectations of one's team is a powerful motivating force. This kind of accountability can unite people to accomplish things they never could on their own. Having the team come to an agreement on how they want to behave is the first step in creating this new context. During this process, the team must also discuss how they will hold each other accountable if someone violates the code. This is an important point: you cannot break the Code of Ethics in holding someone accountable.

We had a CNA in one of our neighborhood teams who was unable or unwilling to live by the code that she and her team had created. As her team held her accountable to what she had agreed to, she became angry and walked off the job. On her way out, she took the signed and framed Code of Ethics off the wall and threw it on the floor, smashing the glass. The team was terribly upset. She had not only disappointed her team, but she had also disrespected their code.

Looking at that incident, I realized that if the traditional structure had been in place in that neighborhood, it might have taken months for the managers to recognize and deal with the poor behavior of this CNA. It is likely she would have stayed working in that community far longer than she did and continued her poor performance. I also recognized that the team had adopted a powerful sense of ownership, so much so that they were incensed when someone disrespected the code they had created together.

Creating that kind of team is not easy, and it takes a lot of time. But when I think about the time that managers spend in dealing with an underperforming employee, I understand and appreciate the power of shifting accountability.

GIVING GRACE

Besides facilitating the shifting of accountability, the guide must teach the self-managed team about the importance of grace. On a team, "I am you, and you are me." Meaning, what happens to you happens to me. This is the philosophy of the Ubuntu culture in action and is completely different from the dog-eat-dog context of the institutional model.

As I have stated previously, we are constantly judging ourselves and others. That kind of judgment causes great harm to a team. On a team, if you point a finger at someone else, you are pointing three fingers at yourself. Religions define grace as the unmerited favor of God. Here, I use the term not as religious vernacular, but as a secular vehicle for expressing how team members care for each other. Instead of passing judgment on each other, the members of a team "give grace" to each other, even if that grace is unwarranted.

While creating peer accountability, a guide must be aware of the dangers of creating a context that is harsh and unforgiving. It is not unusual for people who have never before had a voice to react in a robust way when it comes to holding others accountable.

We are born with a need for equity. If you do not believe me, take two 3-year-olds, pour them each some juice, and watch what happens. If you did not manage to get the level of juice in each glass within a millimeter of each other, you will hear about it. Equity is fairness and impartiality. That sounds good on the surface to most of us. We want things to be fair. But teams can be guilty of applying a "vicious evenhandedness" that can destroy the team (Thomas, personal communication, 2016). Dr. Bill Thomas uses the phrase to describe how the institution treats its elders. I am borrowing it here to describe what can happen in a team bound and determined to make things fair. It is the same thing managers do when they fall into the "lie" of treating everyone the same. If not balanced with grace, evenhandedness can become vicious, mean, and destructive.

Caregiving is an art, and it is impossible to measure the absolute fairness of every action, interaction, task, or job. You cannot measure productivity in a care community like you can in a factory. When we try to reduce the art of caregiving to productivity standards, we forfeit its beauty. It becomes a task rather than the art of deep knowing. Because we are constantly judging others differently than we judge ourselves, it is very easy for teams to cross this line of wanting things to be fair and equitable and throwing people under the bus for "not doing their share." Grace is a beautiful thing on a team. Leaders create a context for success when they teach their teams the importance of "giving grace."

GROWING TRUST

Trust is another context that must be changed to support a new organizational design and a caring community. Trust is the vessel in which a caring community sails. You cannot have community without trust. Institutions are built and operated without trust. However, person-centered leaders understand you cannot be successful unless trust is present and accounted for.

Patrick Lencioni is a consultant and author who has written extensively about building high-functioning teams. If you are venturing on this journey of developing truly self-managed teams, and I hope you are, then I recommend his books, in particular *Overcoming the Five Dysfunctions of a Team: A Field Guide for Leaders, Managers, and Facilitators*. Lencioni believes in teams and writes about their power to set a company apart from its competition. He states,

> I honestly believe that in this day and age of informational ubiquity and nanosecond change, teamwork remains the one sustainable competitive advantage that has been largely untapped. In the course of my career as a consultant to executives and their teams, I can say confidently that teamwork is almost always lacking within organizations that fail, and often present within those that succeed. (Lencioni, 2005, p. 3)

Trust is one of the five team dysfunctions Lencioni writes about; in fact, he identifies trust as the number one dysfunction of teams. Before writing this book, Lencioni had spent the previous 10 years helping companies develop leadership teams. He found that trust was the most important aspect of a team's success, yet it is also the rarest. Most of his work has been in helping teams grow trust.

Lencioni defines trust as vulnerability. He states, "Team members who trust one another learn to be comfortable being open, even exposed, to one another around their failures, weaknesses, even fears" (Lencioni, 2005, p. 14).

Stephen M. R. Covey is another consultant and author who writes about trust. In his book, *The Speed of Trust: The One Thing That Changes Everything*, Covey asserts that trust is the one thing that is "common to every individual, relationship, team, family, organization, nation, economy or civilization," and that if removed would destroy "*the most powerful government, the most successful business, the most thriving economy, the most influential leadership, the greatest friendship, the strongest character, the deepest love*." But he also states that trust, if developed, has "the potential to create unparalleled success and prosperity in every dimension of life" (Covey, 2006, p. 1). Covey contends that trust is a powerful motivator, and despite common beliefs, it is a "pragmatic, tangible, actionable asset that you can create."

So, trust is the most important aspect of a team, and can be developed and grown. Covey gives us a deep understanding of this concept that we used to believe was ambiguous, illusive, and out of our control. I believe that formal leaders can change the context of their communities by growing trust. Although it may take time and patience, growing trust within a team is imperative to the team's success as well as yours.

Only a few care communities have dared to undertake the challenging work of organizational redesign. This type of redesign is built into the Household Model and the Green House® model because it is essential to creating a sustainable care community. We cannot expect people to change their behavior if we do nothing to change the context created by the institutional model. The organizational architecture of the institutional model is one of the biggest culprits for context creation. But it is not the only one.

LESSON 27
Beyond a Just Culture

The single greatest impediment to error prevention in the medical industry is that we punish people for making mistakes.

—Dr. Lucian Leape, professor of health policy

The context created by the institutional model is a malevolent, punitive culture that starts at the Centers for Medicare & Medicaid Services and filters its way down to the charge nurse on the evening shift. It imposes itself into every aspect and action of our work. How could it not? The fear of making a mistake in a culture that expects perfection captures our attention more than anything else. It preys upon our good will and intentions, creating a state of chronic stress in most of us. Who among us is perfect? Who among us has never made a mistake?

As Alexander Pope said, "To err is human." Yet, we have created a context in our care communities that we will be punished if we do make a mistake. We have created a context where our employees live in a state of stress that shuts down their critical thinking. No wonder they make mistakes. As Dr. Leape stated, this expectation of perfection is our greatest impediment to error prevention. Ahh, the irony astounds me.

I attended a conference session given by Dr. Earl Suttle. He suggested that we should start a "Mistake of the Month Award." I love that idea. He also suggested that formal leaders should win the award first (Suttle, 2013). That is brilliant. What better way to show employees that mistakes will no longer be punished? What better way to have everyone learn from one person's mistakes? What better way to show the vulnerability that builds trust?

David Marx is a mechanical engineer and former aircraft design analyst at Boeing. He has become one of the nation's foremost patient safety leaders and coined the term *just culture* to describe the relationship between accountability and safety. Marx knows a lot about how culture influences safety and the roles leaders play in shaping culture. His firm, Outcome Engineering, now spends the majority of its time helping healthcare providers, organizations, and regulators understand modern risk management using the just culture model.

As leaders of care communities, we have a lot to learn from David Marx about changing the context of our communities away from the punitive culture and toward a just culture. In a just culture, employees know that optimal safety is valued. We do not want to make unnecessary mistakes. We do not want to make the same mistake over and over again. But when errors do occur, we see them as learning opportunities. For this to happen, formal leaders must encourage employees to report errors and near misses. They need to acknowledge and reward employees who do report. Remember, we have been habitualized to cover up mistakes. It will take some time to adjust to this new way of thinking. One of the most important parts of just culture is that employees are held accountable for choices, not punished for mistakes. Clear guidance about what is and is not acceptable behavior must accompany this effort.

Just culture also teaches us that mistakes are seldom the fault of the individual. They are usually the fault of the system. If we blame the individual and terminate her, we have not solved the problem. Changing people without changing the system will not solve the problem; the problem will reoccur.

To create a just culture, we must design safe systems and remove opportunities for errors by managing risk. We must perform a root-cause analysis when an error occurs. I have found one of the best ways to do this is to call a team huddle after a mistake is reported. Have the person who made the mistake talk about what happened. Then have the team conduct a root-cause analysis on the spot. The team identifies ways that they can minimize the chances of that mistake reoccurring and puts that new system into place. This must be done without blaming or shaming the person. The team is not looking for what's wrong with the person, but instead identifies flaws in the system. We really do not need to punish people for making mistakes. They usually feel badly enough and are punishing themselves already. Our job is to console them and then turn that mistake into a learning opportunity for everyone.

In a just culture, excellent training and retraining in core competencies and systems are musts. This is a process improvement model by which we manage system performance through outcome data that we share with the team. Most important, leaders must build a supportive structure for when errors occur by training staff to respectfully catch each other's mistakes and correct them.

Through his just culture model, Marx teaches leaders to recognize three different kinds of behavior that we can expect from employees:

1. *Human error:* an inadvertent action; inadvertently doing other than what should have been done; slip, lapse, mistake

2. *At-risk behavior:* a behavioral choice that increases risk where risk is not recognized or is mistakenly believed to be justified

3. *Reckless behavior:* behavioral choice to consciously disregard a substantial and unjustifiable risk

Marx (2007) advises us on how to respond to each of these three different behaviors in a helpful diagram, which I have adapted to reflect possible actions in a care community, to be relevant to our work (see diagram).

I believe this diagram helps us see the distinct differences between human error and choice. It also helps us see the difference between a choice that the employee believes is justified (because the benefit outweighs the risk to a resident), and a choice that disregards the resident's well-being in favor of the employee's convenience. When an employee makes an error, console her and then conduct process improvement. When an employee chooses to take a risk she feels is justified for the benefit of a resident, coach her. When an employee exhibits reckless behavior, then punishment is appropriate.

Let me add that there are times when at-risk behavior can become reckless. If you have already coached an employee on at-risk behavior and removed incentives for repeating that behavior, conducted a root-cause analysis, and proposed other ways of responding when faced with that same situation, then the at-risk behavior has now moved into reckless behavior. For example, if someone is making the same mistake over and over again after you and the team have done a root-cause analysis and fixed any systemic problems, then the mistakes are now a result of the person's inability to perform. A just culture does not mean you never punish people. It simply gives a guide for appropriate accountability. Just culture is not the blame-free culture of La-La Land. It does not absolve you from your responsibility of creating optimal safety. It

Human error	At-risk behavior	Reckless behavior
Product of the current system design	A choice; risk believed insignificant or justified	Conscious disregard of unjustifiable risk
"I forgot her pressure relief cushion. It wasn't in her chair."	*"She requires two people to lift her, but I couldn't find anyone to help me, and she needed to go to the bathroom."*	*"I didn't complete her treatment because it is lengthy and it was nearing the end of my shift. I documented that I had done it."*
Manage through changes in: • Processes • Procedures • Training • Design • Environment	Manage through: • Removing incentives for at-risk behaviors • Creating incentives for healthy behaviors • Increasing situational awareness	Manage through: • Remedial action • Disciplinary action
CONSOLE	COACH	PUNISH

does help you change the context of your community and remove the fear that is inherent in a punitive culture.

UNIVERSAL ACCOUNTABILITY

I believe that just culture is just one more step in creating a new context for a care community, but that we must move beyond just culture to universal accountability, a higher accountability for all of us. It means we each have an important role to play in our community, and with that role comes the following:

- *A voice:* the right to be heard and have our voices become a part of the dialog in which we make decisions as a team or community. This does not mean we always get our way, but that our voices matter.

- *Belonging:* the sense that we are a part of something larger than ourselves and that we matter

- *A responsibility:* to honor and respect each person in our community

- *A responsibility:* to own our emotions and to resolve conflicts that may impede our ability to meet our goals

- *A responsibility:* to contribute and be present, in meetings, learning circles, and huddles that contribute to our success

The institutional model created a context in which only a handful of people hold authority and accountability. Those people then run themselves ragged trying to keep everything in line. In a community, we help each other. In a community with universal accountability, we are each accountable because we each have a voice. We are better as human beings when we work in a community and each of us is accountable.

I often find myself coaching employees by drawing upon this concept of universal accountability. It is a powerful construct for changing the context of our communities. I usually form a question to draw out the understanding of this construct, something like, "Who is responsible for ensuring that our residents have enough staff to provide the care they deserve?" Or "Whose resident [or job] is this?" Of course, the answer is always obvious and the answer is always, "Everyone." As a formal leader, you have to back these kinds of questions up by modeling the behaviors you want. So get out there and show people what universal accountability is by working alongside your employees, and not barking orders from the sidelines. You cannot create universal accountability if you are afraid to get your hands dirty. Accountability begins with you.

FOUR-LEAF CLOVERS

For as long as I have worked in long-term care, there has been a context of managers' settling for less than the best in their employees. Somewhere we bought into the idea that we are the stepchildren of healthcare; that is, we only deserve the leftovers when it comes to attracting and retaining employees. This settling for less than the best has created a context that our elders do not deserve.

My friend and colleague David Farrell writes about Triple Crown winners in *Meeting the Leadership Challenge in Long-Term Care: What You Do Matters*, a book he co-authored with Cathy Brady and Barbara Frank. He defines this type of employee as being competent and reliable and having a great attitude. He outlines a very specific process of determining through your staff roster who are your Triple Crown Winners and who are not. Farrell contends, and I agree, that by settling for people who do not have these characteristics, you are hurting the elders in your community, your staff who are Triple Crown winners, and your organization. You are creating a context where poor performance, especially in the all-important area of relational competence, is tolerated. That creates a context of mediocrity.

I believe that our elders need and deserve to have the very best staff to care for them. Long-term care is not the stepchild of healthcare. It is the epitome of care partnering. It requires the highest level of skills as well as a deep-knowing, an attention to the whole person and her environment. It requires exceptional assessment and clinical skills, for sure, but also the ability to work together across disciplines. We are not treating an illness or injury; our work is the sacred work of creating a care community where everyone can experience well-being. We are the masters of care, not the stepchildren. Hospitals are learning from our experience in person-centered care. They are looking to us to teach them what the Roseto experience has taught us all about social capital and health (Lesson 5).

Understanding this, Vivage communities adopted the Triple Crown winner context. But along the way, we came to realize we needed a fourth expectation of our employees. Yes, we need and want them to be competent, to know their jobs and do them well. We want them to be reliable, to do what they say they will do. We need to be able to count on them. We certainly need them to have great attitudes and the ability to work well with others. In our work, having a great attitude is a part of competence. But we also realized we need and expect them to be accountable. By accountable, we mean to be willing to learn and grow from their mistakes. So, borrowing on Farrell's work, we added accountability to our list of expectations of staff to help our employees become "Four-Leaf Clovers." The same principles apply as with the Triple Crown winners with the additional expectation of holding themselves accountable. As person-centered leaders, we must stop settling for less than the best and begin to help employees become Four-Leaf Clovers. Identify those in your organization who are your Four-Leaf Clovers. You probably could make a list right now off the top of your head. Four-leaf clovers are rare. There is 1 in every 10,000 three-leaf clovers. If you ever find one, legend states that you are going to have some good luck. So you better hang on to it. So it is with your staff. If you have Four-Leaf Clovers, then publicly praise them. Congratulate them. Also find the people who are Three-Leaf Clovers and bring them in individually and congratulate them. Share with them everything wonderful about them, and then tell them you believe in them and know they can become Four-Leaf Clovers. Tell them you are there to help them grow into a Four-Leaf Clover, and then work with them on a growth plan. Check in with them often on their progress toward growing and becoming a Four-Leaf Clover.

Then take a look at your Two-Leaf Clovers, and, if you have any, your One-Leaf Clovers. Ask yourself if you believe they can grow into Four-Leaf Clovers. Give them a chance with growth plans. If they are not willing or able to grow, then the only way you can continue to care for them is by letting them go. You will change the context of your care community beyond a just culture when everyone is on a journey of growth, even you.

100% RESPONSIBILITY

The last construct I want to share with you is the concept of 100% responsibility. There are many self-help gurus who espouse the concept of 100% responsibility in your personal life. But for this purpose, I want to discuss 100% responsibility in terms of working in a team or community. The idea is that on a team or in a community each of us owns and holds 100% responsibility, no more and no less.

We all know what holding less than 100% responsibility looks like. We make judgments about our co-workers who do not carry their 100% all the time. When someone takes less than their 100% responsibility, it impacts the outcome of the whole. In a care community, we rely on each other to manage all of the work that needs to be completed. I often say, "There are no extra people here." We do not have extra people standing around looking for something to do. In our world, everyone is busy and everyone has a hard job. Therefore, it is vital that each of us carry our 100%.

Please notice the difference between carrying your 100% responsibility and equity. Two CNAs can have the same job description. They both work their 8-hour shift without goofing off. They arrive on time, take their breaks, care for their residents, and complete all of their assigned tasks. One of the CNAs is able to care for six elders, and the other cares for seven elders. Can we say that the CNA who cares for seven elders is more productive than the one who cares for six elders? Can we say the one who cares for six elders it taking less than her 100% responsibility? The answers to these questions is no. Caregiving is an art, not a science. It is entirely possible that both CNAs can carry their 100% responsibility.

So what does carrying *less* than your 100% responsibility look like on a team or in a community? Here are a few examples:

- coping quietly, not speaking up when affected
- being unwilling to address conflict
- working on charts during meetings
- not showing up for Huddles or Learning Circles
- always arriving late to avoid making rounds
- blaming others for problems
- using a cell phone during shifts or meetings

There are many other ways that we can take less than our 100% responsibility. When we do that, we are asking our team or co-workers to pick up the slack, and that is truly not fair or equitable.

But this concept of 100% responsibility also recognizes the harm that can come from taking more than your 100% responsibility. I often find this in care communities. When this happens, people are taking on the "hero" or "savior" archetype. We often mistake this kind of behavior as positive. We mistakenly acknowledge the employee who is constantly taking on more than her 100% responsibility because we have done nothing to hold accountable the people who take less than their 100% responsibility. We are grateful someone is taking up the slack. That lets us off the hook with our own responsibility of ensuring everyone is taking their 100% responsibility.

So what does taking *more* than your 100% responsibility look like in a care community? See if you recognize any of these behaviors:

- "I have shown her twice how to do this, and she still is doing it wrong. I will have to do it for her."
- "He did not remember to replace the supplies, so I will do it for him." (And I tell everyone I had to do it because he forgot.)
- "She never completes her work, but I am not going to say anything because she might get mad."

- "I will call everyone on the team and remind them of the deadline."

- "It is easier to do it myself."

- "She always calls in on the weekends, but I know she has a young child, so I am letting it slide."

A person-centered leader can change the context of her community by ensuring that each person holds her 100% responsibility, no more, no less. That is not inconsistent with the need for time-limited special treatment or avoiding a vicious evenhandedness. When you talk about 100% responsibility, it is important that you understand the difference and are able to communicate that difference to your staff. Not doing so will create the dangerous perception that you are not taking your 100% responsibility and are playing favorites.

If we look back to the story of Roscoe Elementary School (Lesson 6), we can see that changing the context of a care community means we must go beyond a just culture. A just culture only rights the wrongs of a punitive culture. Although it is important to right those wrongs, just culture will not get you the kinds of results that Roscoe Elementary School enjoyed. Those kinds of results are available only to the leaders who are able to blend the dialectic of accountability and caring in a supportive way. Those results are for those who dare to elevate everyone in their community to a higher accountability built upon trust and mutual caring. Using the constructs in this lesson will help create that kind of culture. But when it comes to institutional culture, there are more contexts that must also be changed. As organizational gardeners, we must also be aware of the organizational climate.

LESSON 28
Organizational Climate

Over 70% of people leave their jobs because of the way they are led.

—Norman Drummond, minister and leadership coach

Yikes! I am not sure where Norman Drummond got that figure of 70%, but if that is true, we have some work to do, leaders. I am willing to bet that more than 70% of the people reading this book could tell me a story of a time that they were disappointed or even hurt by someone they reported to. My children are blessed at this time in their careers to report to people who understand leadership and use the power of their leadership to create a wonderful climate. That has not always been the case for them. I have reported to leaders who understood organizational climate as well as those who did not. Working for those who did not was a frustrating and sometimes stressful experience. Working for those that did and who adjusted their own behavior to create a warm climate was a joy.

If you are a formal leader, then you are an organizational gardener. Like gardeners of all kinds, you reap what you sow. But unlike other types of gardeners, you have control over the climate. If I were able to give that kind of power to vegetable gardeners, they would have no problem reaping a beautiful harvest. So, I have to ask, "How's the weather?"

Is your organizational climate warm and wonderful, like a tropical island? Or is it cold and harsh, like a winter in Fairbanks, Alaska? Do you even know what your climate is like? If so, how can you tell? Schneider, Ehrhart, and Macey (2013) define organizational climate as "employees' shared perceptions or experiences of the policies, practices, and procedures of their workplace and the behaviors that get rewarded, supported, and expected there" (Schneider, Ehrhart, & Macey, 2013, p. 362). Organizational climate is different from organizational culture. Both are important to understand. If culture is the "cloud" we are all living in, then climate is the temperature that exists within the cloud.

Whereas culture is the way we do things around our community, climate is how we feel about it. Culture is the result of long-held values, norms, rules, and policies. Climate is a short-term phenomenon based upon the beliefs, attitudes, actions, and priorities of the current formal leadership. When my friend David Farrell says, "When you have seen one nursing home, you've seen one nursing home;" he is talking about climate. When I talk about being able to go into any nursing home and find some of the same behaviors, I am talking about culture.

The best example of culture that I can give you is an experience I had on my first visit to Australia. Traveling to Australia from the United States was a 30-hour ordeal. I arrived in Brisbane in the early morning. I was there to conduct several trainings. I knew I only had one day to get on Australia time and be able to function as a facilitator the next morning. To stay awake, I decided to take a stroll around Brisbane. As I was walking down the sidewalk, I kept bumping into people. After a while, this became a little irritating. I was beginning to think that Aussies did not know how to walk down a sidewalk. Then it struck me. In Australia, they drive on the left side of the road, so they walk on the left side of the sidewalk. When they approach someone while walking, they naturally step to the left. Coming from the United States, every time I approached someone along my stroll around Brisbane, I stepped to the right and the Aussies stepped to the left, and we ran into each other. Our cultures were bumping into one another. They did not think about or plan to step to the left. It was not in their conscious thought. It just happened. And the same goes for my behavior. That is culture; it is everything we do without thinking about it or planning it.

Organizational climate is also a subconscious act, unless the leaders are completely self-aware and intentional about creating a climate in which people want to work.

The Eden Alternative philosophy asserts that there is a "warmth continuum" along which every care community falls. Eden characterizes warm organizations as "optimistic, trusting, and generous," and cold organizations as "pessimistic, cynical, and stingy" (Certified Eden Associate Training Educator's

Guide, 2015). Where does your organization fall along the warmth continuum, and why does it matter?

Numerous studies have found positive relationships between warm organizational climates and various measures of organizational success, most notably for metrics such as staff retention, productivity, customer satisfaction, and profitability:

- Denison (1990) found that an organizational climate that encourages employee involvement and empowerment in decision making predicts the financial success of the organization.

- Schneider (1996) found that service and performance climates predict customer satisfaction.

- Potosky and Ramakrishna (2001) found that an emphasis on learning and skill development was significantly related to organizational performance.

- Ekvall (1996) found a positive relationship between organizational climates that emphasize creativity and innovation and their profits.

- Thompson (1996) found that companies using progressive human resource practices to impact climate, such as customer commitment, communication, empowerment, innovation, rewards and recognition, community involvement/ environmental responsibility, and teamwork, outperformed organizations with less progressive practices. (ERC, 2014)

If you are engaging in cultural transformation, understanding organizational climate is a priority. Gardeners cannot grow a garden in a cold, frozen climate. Likewise, without the advantages of a warm climate, one that is optimistic, trusting, and generous, sustainable change is impossible. The great news here is that formal leaders control the climate. It is important to know where your organization falls along the warmth continuum. The Eden Alternative offers tools that measure organizational warmth (http://www.edenalt.org/resources/warmth-surveys/). An important caveat: do not confuse organizational climate with employee satisfaction. Although having a warm climate can contribute to employee satisfaction, they are two different things. Climate assessments measure optimism, trust, and generosity, not satisfaction.

In my work, we often conduct on-site climate assessments. We understand the importance of leadership in our world. The minute we start to see a negative trend in outcomes or we receive calls from a number of disgruntled employees, we know we need to assess the climate. Anytime we take on a new consulting project or consider the management of a care community, we conduct operational, clinical, and organizational climate and culture assessments. My team and I will spend time in the community speaking with as many stakeholders as we can. From these interviews, we identify potential culture or climate problems that need to be addressed.

You can have the best operational and clinical systems in the world, but if they are not a part of a warm, supportive climate, they will not be effective. We are a business for people by people. A context of optimism, trust, and generosity is the foundation for good systems and best practices to be applied.

There is one funny aspect about climate I want you to be aware of. Formal leaders usually believe that the climate in their organization is warmer than the employees perceive it to be. Using an Eden Alternative "warmth survey" or, even better, hiring an outside consultant to conduct a climate assessment of your community can give you a realistic picture of your organization's climate. This can be a valuable management tool you can use to gain self-awareness and begin to shift your beliefs, attitudes, actions, and priorities if you find you are working in a cold climate. If you just want a quick and dirty climate analysis, just have someone your staff does not know come in and walk around your community, listening to the conversations. Climate is the feel of the organization. You can feel the warmth or the cold of any organization if you "tune into" it.

A word of caution about culture and climate assessments: it is often hard for formal leaders to hear the perceptions others have of them. We think of ourselves as warm, caring, and compassionate people. Others may not perceive us that way. Just as it is hard for managers to hear growth opportunities from their consultants, hearing how your employees perceive you and the workplace can be traumatizing. It is not fun, but it is important that you listen and respond appropriately as well as thank them for their feedback. Then you go to work changing the context so that those negative perceptions start to change. Remember, sometimes growth is painful.

Another unusual aspect of organizational climate is that change consumes warmth. As you introduce more and more change into your community, it will start to "cool off," unless you are constantly applying warming techniques. One of the best of these is listening, really listening, to your staff. Then support them in solving the problems they feel are important. Do not give them the answers; act as the facilitator and resource bearer so they can solve their own problems. Learning circles are a great way of listening (Lesson 30). Everything else I have discussed in this book is a climate warming technique. Start changing the context by warming the climate, and watch the magic start to happen.

The only risk-free human environment is a coffin.

—Dr. William Thomas, co-founder of The Eden Alternative

"Safety above all else" has been the mantra of care communities for decades under current regulations. Born out of an unfortunate history of insufficient safety, this mantra resounds daily in our ears and hearts. This context is reinforced through federal regulatory deficiencies, such as the loathed F323, failure to prevent accidents. That regulation has always concerned me because an accident by its very definition is "a sudden event that is not planned or intended and that causes damage or injury" (Merriam-webster.com).

It is, therefore, an oxymoron to cite a care community for failure to prevent something that is unplanned or unintended. This goes beyond the expectation of perfection. This takes us into the realm of psychics. I remember walking directly behind my grandmother when one of her dogs ran between her legs and caused her to fall and break her pelvis. I was right behind her. I saw it happen, but I could not do anything about it. It was an accident. The regulators might say she should not have had her dogs running loose in the house. The problem with that kind of "surplus safety" is that it does not account for the upside of risk.

The phrase *surplus safety* was coined by Dr. Bill Thomas and Dr. Judah Ronch, dean of the Erickson School of Aging at the University of Maryland, Baltimore County. It describes the current institutional context surrounding risk. Thomas and Ronch define risk as the possibility of an unanticipated outcome. Our current context sees only the downside of risk, but Thomas and Ronch remind us that there is also an upside of risk. Our lives are worth living because we enjoy the opportunity to experience this upside of risk every day. Through our fear of regulatory fines or litigation, however, we have removed the opportunity for our residents to experience upside risk.

My grandmother enjoyed the upside of risk when she had animal companions in her house. She believed that was more important to her well-being than the downside risk of having one of them run between her legs and trip her. I live in a state, Colorado, whose economy depends upon upside risk. There are people from all over the country who travel to this fine state each winter. They venture up to the top of steep mountains in subfreezing temperatures, strap two pieces of lumber on their feet, and hurl themselves down icy slopes, all in the quest of upside risk. No one ever publishes how many people die in these ventures annually, but the risk is real.

Many of our residents come to us because their families cannot keep them safe at home. Somehow, we are supposed to keep them from falling, when, in fact, they fall much more in care communities than they do at home. All of this is to point out that surplus safety is not the context for well-being. It led us to restrain residents to prevent them from falling. It led to the implementation of chair and bed alarms, which have been proven to cause more falls than prevent them. It led us to over-administer psychotropic medications to residents. It has created the barbaric practice of waking up elders every 2 hours to turn them in their beds. This sleep fragmentation is a form of torture that our military uses to get prisoners of war to talk. It prevents the human brain from entering into the healing stages of sleep. Yet, we perform this particular type of torture on hundreds of thousands of elders nightly across this country. Surplus safety has also led to other fear-based practices that interfere with the well-being of our residents and staff. There are, frankly, too many to mention.

I remember one particular example of surplus safety an administrator in Colorado shared with me during a phone call. She told me that "the state" had just left her building and that the surveyors were contemplating citing her community for having a potluck dinner. Families and staff each brought favorite dishes to share. This particular ritual occurs in every care community across the country because it is one that everyone enjoys. I could imagine other phone lines lighting up around the country as culture change pioneers were calling each other outraged over this potential citation. I am sure those surveyors had returned to their offices to ask for guidance, and that the state regulators were calling their federal counterparts, trying to get a determination.

Fortunately, the Centers for Medicare & Medicaid Services is on the side of residents and their rights. They want to promote person-centered care and all of its advantages to the well-being of elders. But they also have a responsibility, just as we do, to ensure the safety of elders as much as possible. On this day, the rights of the elders were maintained, and surplus safety was traded for optimal safety. The determination came down—let them have potluck! The state regulators had determined that as long as the community gave residents the option of eating a meal prepared in the kitchen or sharing in the potluck, the community could continue to hold potlucks.

Thomas and Ronch want us to know that when we remove all risk from life, we remove the reason for living. Surplus safety crushes the human spirit and can actually harm our elders. We would never consider preventing a child from walking or riding a bicycle or engaging in any other activity that might pose a risk but that could help his development. Why would we condemn an elder to a lack of opportunity for development that comes from removing risks? For more on this topic, visit The Eden Alternative website (Surplus Safety: When Can Safety Harm Us? www.edenalt.org/ondemandwebinar/surplus-safety-can-safety-harm-us/).

Optimal safety is the new context and requires more from leaders of care communities, just as growing a sustainable care community requires more than operating an institution. It requires us to not fall into fear and resort to surplus safety. When I was working as an administrator, I had a resident who had been placed in our community by adult protective services, who believed she was unsafe at home. Despite the fact that she had set on fire the trailer she and her husband lived in with her husband in it, she was an active participant and decision maker in her life. Her husband had purchased a new trailer and parked it across a very busy interstate highway near our community. Most days, he would ride his bicycle to the community, get something to eat, and then the two of them would venture back to their trailer. Every day I said a little prayer as I watched them traverse the busy street, heading home. She eventually was able to return home permanently and resume her normal life. A few years later, she gave a concert in town that I was able to attend. As I sat there, it occurred to me that had I been a harbinger of fear, she might not be living a full and abundant life. She might never have had a chance to return to her home.

Had she been placed in an institutional home instead of one on the journey toward person-centered care, her spirit might have withered and died.

Creating a context of optimal safety does not mean you take unnecessary or unmanaged risks. Before letting this woman leave our grounds, we had assessed her ability to safely walk to her home and asked her husband to accompany her. We repeated that assessment quarterly to ensure her continued capacity. Because we knew the fire happened because she had not been taking her medications, we made sure that her medications were prescribed at times when she would be in our community so we could carefully monitor her behavior. We also had the piano tuned for her so she could practice. (They did not have one in her trailer.) She brought her dog to live with her, and he also accompanied the couple as they walked home. We met with her daughter, her case manager, her husband, and the woman herself to carefully document her wishes as well as our shared agreements that she would leave and return each day during times that did not coincide with heavy traffic. We also agreed that if she could not get back to the community on time or if she was too tired to walk, she would call us and we would come get her. All of that effort created a context of optimal safety that allowed her the opportunity for upside risk without putting the community into unmitigated downside risk. Would it have been better to just tell her no because of the risk?

Optimal safety requires some shared risk on the part of the elder and the community that is responsible for her safety. It requires a lot more work and attention to managing risk so that it does not become downside risk. It also requires a lot of education and changing the beliefs of your staff. Surplus safety has been ingrained in their hearts, and those hearts break anytime an elder is hurt. Staff do not ever want to be the cause of an elder getting hurt. They do not want to be blamed for it, certainly. But more than that, they cannot stand to see an elder in pain. Teaching them about the dangers of surplus safety is a prerequisite for changing that context.

You cannot achieve person-centered care in a surplus safety context. I know that I rest my head easily on my pillow at night knowing that we did everything we could to help this elder and the many others who lived in our community to not fall prey to the callous punishment of surplus safety. I hope you will, as well.

Formal leaders are the context creators. You set the climate of your community, and you set the context for all behavior through your values, actions, and priorities. The beautiful thing is that if you do not like the current context, you can change it by changing your behavior. The solution to creating a caring community is creating a new context through organizational redesign, moving beyond a just culture to universal accountability and 100% responsibility, assessing your climate, and creating optimal safety.

Through shifting beliefs and changing the context, you are on a certain path toward sustainable person-centered care. Now you just need to replace some routines that continue to shape a culture you do not want or like.

CHAPTER 8

Solving the Problem

Replacing Routines

Keystone Habits

Good habits are worth being fanatical about.

—John Irving, author

Often I hear how formal leaders feel overwhelmed with how to bring culture change to their communities. It all just seems so big. With everything leaders already have to attend to, how would they possibly be able to make these changes? So they spend a lot of time planning for these large events or strategies to "change the culture" of their community. They spend a lot of time planning, but there never seems to be enough time to implement the plan. That is when they say things like, "We will begin our culture change journey when we are fully staffed." Or even better, "We are in survey window now. We will begin after our survey."

The problem with these statements is that you will never be fully staffed until you create a new way. And the surveyors are always coming. They are either in your community or coming soon. Count on it. The faster you begin this journey, the less often the surveyors will be coming. The system is broken. Admit it, and do something differently. It does not have to be a big life-changing event. You do not have to introduce open dining or self-managed teams or train every person in your community overnight. You just have to begin. Now the question becomes, "Where do I begin?"

In their book, *Switch: How to Change Things When Change Is Hard*, Chip Heath and Dan Heath show us how successful changes follow a pattern, a pattern you can use to make the changes that matter to you, whether you want to change the world or change your care community. The Heaths bring together decades of research in psychology and sociology, among other fields, to give us a pathway to transformative change.

The Heaths draw on the metaphor of the rider and the elephant that I introduced in Lesson 15 from Haidt's book, *The Happiness*

Hypothesis. To remind you, the rider is the conscious, rational, thinking part of our brains, and the elephant is the subconscious, emotional, intuitive part. The "formula" that the Heaths share with us is fairly simple (Heath & Heath, 2010):

1. Direct the rider,

2. Motivate the elephant,

3. Shape the path.

I encourage you to read this fascinating book. For my purposes, however, I want to point out two of the pathways in this book that can help us understand how to begin this important journey. The first of these is one step in directing the rider. The Heaths call it "script the critical moves." When the problem is big, like the transformation of a care community's decades-long culture, our tendency is to think that the solution has to be just as big. When the solution is too big, the elephant takes over. When the elephant takes over, the rider gets tired. Remember the research that shows that our willpower is like a muscle? When emotions are running high, as they will in a change effort that is too big, the elephant charges and the rider muscle gets worn out.

When we script the critical moves, we are directing the rider toward exactly which routines we want him to replace. We take the lofty goal of changing the culture of an organization and boil it down to the very specific goal of replacing that routine with a new one.

The next is the idea that we are confusing what we perceive as resistance to change with lack of clarity. If the elephant does not understand exactly where the rider wants him to go, if the path is unclear, the elephant will resist. The root cause of that resistance is not a dislike of change. It is the absence of clarity. Uncertainty causes anxiety. When we shrink the change, we calm the elephant and make the change clear and doable. Shrinking the change also gives us small wins that then fuel the energy we need to create more change (Heath & Heath, 2010).

So, where do we begin? Which routine do we replace first? What are those critical moves that will help us shape a transformational journey?

In his book, *The Power of Habit: Why We Do What We Do in Life and Business,* Charles Duhigg introduces us to the concept of "keystone habits," which are those habits that have a ripple effect in changing other habits. As Duhigg points out, "Some habits matter more than others in remaking businesses and lives. . . . Keystone habits start a process that, over time, transforms everything" (Duhigg, 2012, p. 100).

To illustrate the power of keystone habits in transforming a company, Duhigg recounts the story of Alcoa's dramatic turnaround in the late 1980s at the hands of a new CEO, Paul O'Neill. Although many people, including investors and managers, considered O'Neill's approach to be foolish in light of Alcoa's shrinking profits, O'Neill understood what they did not. Namely, some habits have the power to "start a change reaction" that will begin to disrupt many other habits throughout the organization. He also understood some of the workings of the brain. He knew that he would not be able to force people to change. So, instead he attacked one habit. At the time of O'Neill's hiring, Alcoa was not only losing market share and profitability, but also dealing with a terrible safety record. At that time, almost every Alcoa plant in the country was enduring at least one employee accident every week. While the stockholders expected the new CEO to focus on profitability and market share, O'Neill focused instead on worker safety. They thought he was crazy.

O'Neill's background as a middle manager in the U.S. Department of Veterans Affairs, combined with his obsession with making lists, gave him experience in recognizing institutional habits. These were routines so ingrained in the organization that they were imbedded firmly in the subconscious mind. When that happens, O'Neill says, "We are basically ceding decision-making to a process that occurred without actually thinking." Researchers have discovered these kinds of "institutional habits" in almost every organization or company they have studied.

What amazes me is that almost every nursing home shares some of the same institutional habits, despite being populated with completely different people. What O'Neill understood is just how dangerous these habits are. So, when he was searching for which keystone habit to use in turning Alcoa around, he knew he needed something that everyone would agree was important.

How can you argue with worker safety? Using that keystone habit, he was fulfilling his employee's well-being need for security. He was also disrupting the routines that were automatic across all of Alcoa's plants. Through that process of replacing one routine, he changed many others.

Using worker safety as his focus, O'Neill brought all of the constituencies together. The workers certainly appreciated this effort, and so did the unions. The managers quickly followed suit because O'Neil required them to report directly to him within 24-hours of a worker injury. The only managers who received promotions were those who complied with these new directives. The only way a unit president could report to O'Neill within 24 hours of an accident occurring was to hear from his vice president. Vice presidents, therefore, had to be in constant communication with their floor managers. And floor managers had to build strong relationships with their workers and encourage them to report problems as soon as they noticed them. Workers were encouraged to identify potential areas for improving their own safety, so they felt empowered. This one keystone habit caused a complete redesign of communication systems at Alcoa. It also began to dismantle the hierarchy.

As they began to experience small wins, other aspects of the company started to change, as well. The unions, once resistant to every idea coming from management, began to embrace ideas that could improve worker safety, such as measuring the productivity of individual workers. Those measurements could identify flaws in the system, putting safety at risk. Policies that empowered workers, previously fought against by managers, were now embraced because they would help prevent an accident.

Other than saving on worker's compensation losses, one might not imagine that focusing on worker safety could have a large impact on profitability. That was not the case at Alcoa. During O'Neill's tenure, and prior to his stint as George W. Bush's Secretary of Treasury, Alcoa made a dramatic turnaround. By the time he left Alcoa, the company's annual net income had increased five-fold. That is the power of keystone habits and a leader willing to stick with them to change an organization. O'Neill had to endure skepticism to fulfill his belief in keystone habits (Duhigg, 2012).

Duhigg reminds us that

small wins are exactly what they sound like, and are part of how keystone habits create widespread changes. A huge body of research has shown that small wins have enormous power, an influence disproportionate to the accomplishments of the victories themselves. . . . Once a small win has been accomplished, forces are set in motion that favor another small win. Small wins fuel transformative changes by leveraging tiny advantages into patterns that convince people that bigger achievements are within reach. (Duhigg, 2012, p. 112)

Keystone habits help you as a leader to direct the path by scripting the moves. They also help you motivate the elephant by shrinking the change. Let us begin to identify those keystone habits that will change a care community by identifying habits we can all agree are important. When I look for the common denominators in a care community, I always think of our elders. We all love our residents. They are the common denominator that feeds our elephants. If we can find a keystone habit that would make their lives better, we would all agree on that.

Another thing we can agree on is ethical principles. It is very hard to argue with doing what is right, proper, and good. It is difficult to find someone who would fault you for doing the right thing, for fairness or equity.

Finally, we can all agree that we need to care about each other, not just the residents. We are caring people. It does not make sense that we would beat each other up. It is not right that we would target each other. We have enough people trying to find fault with us. We need to stick together.

Using these shared agreements, I have identified the keystone habits that I believe will dramatically change a care community. If you will replace these routines, you will immediately begin to see some small wins. Those small wins will energize your community and begin a domino effect that will drive other changes. You can begin all of these today. They all will have a huge difference in the culture and climate of your communities, and they do not cost a penny.

ELDERS AS THE DRIVERS: DAILY COMMUNITY MEETINGS

We can all agree that the elders deserve to have a voice in their community. The institutional model created for us a very strange world that was not shaped by the people who live there but by the people who work there. We can begin to right that wrong by replacing one routine. Daily community meetings were introduced to the culture change movement by an amazing couple who continue to promote the rights of elders to have a voice in shaping their communities. Through their Live Oak Institute, Barry and

Daily Community Meetings

Agenda

Welcoming
- Provides opportunity to connect with the elders before the meeting
- Helps participants feel known and appreciated
- Lets participants know the meeting will begin soon
- Provides opportunity to introduce visitors and guests

Exercises
- Helps participants become more alert for the meeting
- Increases health and well-being
- Provides a learning experience for individuals and group

Opening Song
- Connects people to one another
- Builds group spirit and joy

Community News
- Introduction of new community members (staff and elders)
- Announcements (coming events and past events)
- Life events for participants and their families
- Planning and decision making

World News
- Stimulates and challenges participants
- Invites involvement in community affairs and current topics of national and world discussion

Discussion of the Day
- Stimulates and challenges participants (talking, feeling, and thinking about a topic)
- Helps participants get to know each other
- Provides a point of connection for future conversations
- Encourages problem solving as a community

Closing Song
- Lets people know meeting is over
- Gives everyone a good feel for and connection to the group

Deborah Barkan have given us an incredible tool to bring those voices forward. Daily community meetings are just that, an opportunity each day to bring the community together, share with each other, listen to our elders, and engage in community building. The elders should decide the best time for these meetings. Staff should attend, but the meetings ideally should be run by the elders. The Barkans have given us an agenda for these meetings, but your elders could shape their own. Meetings usually last about 30 minutes. These replace the monthly Resident Council meetings, so minutes should be kept. Every day, the residents of the care community are shaping the rhythm of their day, identifying areas for improvement and enjoying community together. As the residents identify areas of improvement, the staff can then immediately conduct a root-cause analysis and implement action plans. Using this forum, complaints are identified and mitigated daily, before they can fester and grow. In one of our communities, our residents told state surveyors that they could leave because all of their issues were being addressed by the staff. They did not need the surveyors interfering in their community. The home did not receive any deficiencies that year.

My organization, Vivage Senior Living, was asked to take over temporary management of a community in Colorado that was in trouble. I will not go into the specifics, but there were some horrific things happening at this home. On the first day of our contract, our newly assigned administrator implemented daily community meetings. One of the elders commented, "This is the first time I have been treated as a human being."

LEARNING CIRCLES AND HUDDLES

My friend LaVrene Norton, founder and executive leader of Action Pact, introduced the culture change movement to one its most valuable tools: the "learning circle." This has the power to dramatically change your care community. The learning circle is taught in almost every training on person-centered care, yet I continually find communities failing to use it. I have struggled to understand why. It may be because the concept of a learning circle is so simple that people cannot conceive how it could make a difference. Or it could be because people cannot find enough chairs. Maybe people do not believe they have any communication challenges in their community. Or maybe it is because it initially makes people feel uncomfortable. One of the hardest things for leaders to do is shut up, to ask the question and then be quiet. Listening may be too hard for some leaders to endure. Whatever reason is preventing you from implementing learning circles in your community, please identify it and fix it.

Learning circles have been around for centuries. There is archeological and anthropological evidence that human beings have been meeting in circle to discuss, plan, resolve conflict, and find the wisdom of the group for a long, long time. Sure, maybe that was because we sat around a fire to keep warm, but there's a power to the circle. There's power in coming together as a community and listening to each other.

Margaret Wheatley, one of my favorite authors, once wrote,

> In my own work, I've been advocating conversation as the means to restore hope for the future. This is as simple as I can get. I've seen that there's no more powerful way to initiate significant change than to convene a conversation. When a community of people discovers that they share a concern, change begins. There is no power equal to a community discovering what it cares about. (Wheatley, 2010)

Wheatley gets it. Just because something is not complicated does not mean it is not powerful. Learning circles are simple and effective. If the problem is that you cannot find enough space or chairs, then stand up in a huddle, but be sure to use the same rules of the learning circle. The rules are there for a reason: to improve our communication. Often people tell me they are not using learning circles, they are using huddles. When I question them about their huddles, I discover they have missed the point completely. The point of a learning circle, or for that matter a huddle, is to abate the problems we naturally have in our communication.

Human beings are really terrible at communication. Any formal leader who says she does not have a problem with communication in her community is wearing blinders. If we became masters of communicating with each other, most of the problems in the world would go away. You are not trying to run the world, but to create a caring community. You need to improve the way people communicate in your community.

Learning circles level us. They remove the barriers of hierarchy that exist in any group of people and that run rampant in our care communities. In the learning circle, we all have an equal voice. Learning circles also mitigate the problem of people who talk too much and people who talk too little or who never talk. They balance us. Learning circles can prevent the "meeting after the meeting" (i.e., the meeting where the people who did not speak up now speak up). The people who were busy talking in the regular meeting, however, are not listening in the "meeting after the meeting." If we are all participating and listening in a meeting, we do not need the "meeting after the meeting."

Learning circles are a keystone habit. They must become the way we now communicate. If you are unfamiliar with learning circles or huddles, an explanation of both is included at the end of this lesson (see "The Learning Circle," "Using the Learning Circle," and "Huddles"). If you know about learning circles and huddles and are not using them daily, please begin today.

A COHESIVE LEADERSHIP TEAM

Leadership is a powerful force. It has the ability to change people's lives or to destroy them. Do not ever discount the power of your position, and use it wisely. Being wise leaders means that you must be consistent in your message. You must become one voice in leading your care community. You must foster and model a high-trust team that cares for each other. That effort must become intentional and consistent. If not, then like children playing their parents against one another, the hands-on staff will divide and conquer. They will wait you out. They have done it before. Many of them have continued their old ways, knowing that the administrator or director of nursing (DON) will only be there a short time. Then another one will come, and they will wait her out as well.

It has been my experience that those communities that manage to create sustainable person-centered care are blessed with leaders who stay more than the average tenure of an administrator or DON. They stay, and during their tenure they work to build a high-functioning cohesive leadership team.

I have witnessed care communities where the formal leaders are stabbing each other in the back. It is not a pretty sight. It creates a context of gossip, fear, uncertainty, and distrust. Hands-on employees mimic the leaders' behaviors. Pretty soon, you have a context of nastiness that bleeds over onto the elders. They do not deserve that.

If you are true to your commitment to bring about transformational change, an essential keystone habit is to grow a team of formal leaders who care for each other and who become one voice in the community. That requires effort. It just does not happen. Formal leadership teams must meet at least 8 hours per month as a team. This meeting should not be about conducting the business of the organization. This meeting is to grow as a high-trust, high-functioning team of leaders. You can meet for 2 hours each week, 4 hours every other week, or a full 8 hours monthly; it does not matter. What matters is that you devote this time to developing as a team.

If I walk into your care community and talk to the activity director, I should know that what she is telling me is the same thing the administrator would tell me. If the DON is out of the building and I talk to the minimum data set coordinator, she should be able to tell me what the DON would. If I am a hands-on caregiver and I need help, I should know that I can talk to any manager and get the same support my own manager would give me. I guarantee if you make the investment in the work of developing a cohesive leadership team, there will be nothing that you cannot do. Make it one of your keystone habits.

These three keystone habits, daily community meetings, learning circles or huddles, and leadership team development, will be powerful ways to begin your journey. They give the elders a voice, they give everyone an equal voice, and they unify the voices of the leadership team. You will very quickly begin to see the small wins they will bring to your community, but you cannot stop there.

Unlike Alcoa, which makes aluminum, you are in the business of creating a caring community. I wish there was only one keystone habit that could do that. But the institutional model has left such a huge scar on our communities that you will need to replace more routines than just these three.

In the last lesson, I discuss some more keystone habits that must be put into place. All of these will begin to dramatically alter the ethos of your community. They will right the wrongs that have been allowed to happen in care communities everywhere. These are the next routines that must be replaced to create a truly caring community.

The Learning Circle

The learning circle gives us an ongoing means to break down the hierarchy. It is through the continued, daily use of this simple tool that we leave the old culture behind. Remember, our culture is our collective habits. Old habits are broken by creating new habits.

Goal: To develop common ground and mutual respect among the diversity of the care community's residents, staff, families, management, departments, shifts, and professions.

Rules for the Learning Circle

- *Everyone sits in a circle* without tables or other obstructions blocking their view of one another.

- *One person is the facilitator* to pose the question or issue. (The question and facilitator may have been determined ahead of time by the team/individual planning the circle. If a universally negative response to a question is predicted, consider shaping the question into two parts. For example: "Share one thing that worries you and one thing that excites you about . . . ")

- *Be aware that emotional topics can be overwhelming* in large circles. If the facilitator believes a question will elicit strong feelings of sadness, depression, grief, or anger, limit the number of participants to between 8 and 10 and keep them apprised of the time allotted for the circle so they may adjust themselves emotionally. Keep the time per person fairly short (30 seconds is good). Remember you will be opening it up for discussion immediately after, and it does not take too long to share the *feeling.*

- *The facilitator poses the question or issue and asks for a volunteer.* A volunteer in the circle responds with his or her thoughts on the chosen topic. The person sitting to the right or left of the first respondent goes next, followed one by one around the circle until everyone has spoken on the subject without interruption.

- *No cross talk or negative body language.* The facilitator should have made this rule clear at the beginning so that they do not need to interrupt often to enforce the rule of no talking across the circle. (Involuntary laughter and simple words of empathy should not be quelled. But others may not add their thoughts or opinions on an issue until it is their turn to speak.)

- *One may choose to pass* rather than to speak when their time comes. But after everyone else in the circle has had their turn, the facilitator goes back to those who passed and allows each another opportunity to respond. Of course, no one is forced to speak, but there is the expectation that they will.

- *Open general discussion* on the topic after everyone has had a chance to speak.

Using the Learning Circle

Learning circles are appropriate for practically any gathering, meeting, or event, including care plan meetings, team meetings, family nights, committee meetings, elder meetings, educational sessions, and information sharing. They can be effective for planning, problem solving, resolving conflict, discussing issues, learning new information, and growing team and community—essentially any situation that requires good communication. Learning circles should be ongoing, regular meetings of the same participants, but they may also be spontaneously organized to deal with a specific issue.

Learning circles can be used to strengthen bonds and create a sense of equality among elders, caregivers, managers, and family members. Participants learn and appreciate that they are all in this together, working to create the world in which to live, work, and grow.

Learning circles convened regularly among teams can heal minor irritations before they develop into seemingly unsolvable problems. Communication lines remain open. Respect among individuals and a sense of community are fostered.

When

Anytime people come together

Team meetings

Neighborhood meetings

Daily elder meetings

Care plan meetings

Committee meetings

Employee education

New employee welcoming

Family meetings

Shift-to-shift reports

Community meetings

Quality improvement meetings

Change of condition meeting

Survey exit conference

Event planning

(continued)

(continued)

Who

Elders

Caregivers

Managers

Families

Volunteers

Team members

Medical director

Therapists

Ombudsmen and surveyors

Why

To begin or end a meeting

To build community

To begin a discussion

To create a safe place

To resolve conflict

To plan

To solve problems

To break down the hierarchy

To level and balance

To give each individual a voice that is heard

To remove the trappings of power

Huddles

In some instances during the work day, it may be burdensome or even impossible to find a space for people to sit to hold a learning circle. In these cases, a huddle can be useful instead. Huddles can be spontaneous and can be held almost anywhere. A huddle is a "stand-up" learning circle. All of the rules of the learning circle should be adhered to, so that you are leveling the hierarchy and balancing voices.

Huddles are a very effective way to engage everyone in problem solving, brain-storming solutions, and care planning for change in an elder's condition (a fall or other incident). Huddles can also be used to adjust to changes in assignments or schedules (e.g., someone goes home sick and needs help with a resident). Huddles allow the team to become very flexible and able to respond to changes quickly.

The Trappings of Power

In order to level the hierarchy, we must be constantly mindful of the trappings of the institutional culture and the old ways of doing things. Who has the power in these situations?

A nurse behind the nurses' station or a family member leaning on the station talking with the nurse?

An elder sitting in her wheelchair or the CNA looking down at her?

A CNA or nurse in uniform standing and talking with an elder who is also standing?

A group of people sitting around a rectangular table?

The Importance of Balance

In a typical work environment, some people do most of the talking. Other people do most of the listening. The learning circle gives the listeners a chance to speak and the talkers a chance to listen. The feelings and opinions of all are important. The learning circle promotes listening skills among all who participate. It allows everyone to have a say without interruption or criticism.

Frequently in situations where the "listeners" are not heard by the "talkers," a phenomenon called "the meeting after the meeting" takes place, creating a scenario in which communication is further broken down, an aura of distrust is fostered, and misinformation and assumptions are perpetuated. It can be a very destructive practice that undermines the progress of the team.

LESSON 31
From Animosity to Reciprocity

Stand up in the presence of the elderly, and show respect for the aged.

—Leviticus 19:32

Have you noticed something very odd in your community? Have you noticed how your staff treat the residents? Have you noticed how they treat each other? Do you not find that odd? I do. How can the same people who care so deeply and give so much of themselves to the residents turn around and be so mean to each other?

Previously, we learned about our tendency to form tribes or constituencies and how those constituencies will battle with each other. As I followed the 2016 U.S. presidential election, I heard so much about the two tribes, Republicans and Democrats, and their nasty treatment of each other. I understand it is in our nature to form these tribes and do battle. It does not make it any more pleasant to watch. I could turn off the television and ignore it. Your elders cannot. In fact, they are at the mercy of the animosity your employees have toward one another. They are the victims of it. And it is up to you to stop the bleeding. Consider this, please. Imagine for just one moment that something has befallen you and you wake up living in your care community. You are now dependent upon someone else for your most basic needs. One of those people that you are now dependent upon walks into your room angry. How do you feel? Uncertain? Concerned? Scared? Is that acceptable?

The sad story is that this has been happening in care communities since they have existed, and leaders are not doing anything about it. It is time now to replace this routine behavior, animosity, with a keystone habit of reciprocity.

GRANDMOTHER'S HOUSE

I hope that you are fortunate enough to have or to have had a grandmother who loved you unconditionally, and who also had the highest expectations of you. I certainly was. My children had that benefit as well. While embraced in that love, I learned about manners and how to be respectful of others. I learned how to share and how to speak to adults. I learned about being kind and forgiving. Grandmother's house was a place of wisdom and a higher accountability.

When we went to Grandmother's house, there were higher standards for our behavior, our language, and our dress. We did not complain about that higher accountability; we just understood it. We understood that we acted in a way to honor our Grandmother. We showed our respect for her station in our family by cleaning up our act, using our manners, and controlling our behavior. My children had the same experience with their Grandmothers. They never complained about it, because they knew if they did not act in a certain way, Grandmother would let them know they were out of line.

You are blessed to work in what is essentially Grandmother's house. As a formal leader in Grandmother's house, you and your entire leadership team must model that higher accountability through your actions, your language, and your dress. But it must not stop there. Your leadership team must bring the elders (Grandmothers and Grandfathers) together and ask them to help you create a code of conduct for Grandmother's house. Every person who enters your community must be taught the Code of Conduct at Grandmother's house. Then you must hold yourself and others accountable to that code.

We can no longer tolerate an ethos that does not honor and respect our elders. They are unable to hold you, your staff, or even their family members to that higher accountability, so now it is your job. Grandmother's house is no place for fighting, back-biting, or anger. It is the place where we are on our best behavior. Our elders deserve that.

Codes of conduct do not have to be lengthy or hard to remember. They should set the standard for behavior at Grandmother's house.

Ones I have used effectively are simple and brief so that everyone can remember them. For example:

- Everyone will be respectful of everyone at all times.

- Everyone will be willing to grow.

- Everyone will be honest.

A new ethos is demanded by the new world you want to create, that begins by changing our most basic behavior. Once your codes have been developed, educate everyone on them. Put them in your inquiry and admissions packets. Include them in your new hire packets. Post them around your community. Remind people of them in your in-services and at family events. We must break the routines of the past that allowed this kind of bad behavior to be tolerated and set a standard of higher expectations for everyone. You will not test your mettle of being a person-centered leader until you have had to hold a family member or your CEO to the Code of Conduct at Grandmother's house. You can remind them that the elders created this and this is their home.

MANAGING CONFLICT

Setting the Code of Conduct for Grandmother's house is just the first step in creating a new ethos that honors your elders. The next, more challenging step is just as vital: mastering the art of managing conflict. I have noticed that in most of our care communities, we have been doing this all wrong. It makes sense. We are all caring people, and we want to fix things for people. We want to help.

Unfortunately, a common scenario plays out daily in most care communities. One of your most valued employees comes to your office to complain about another employee. You listen intently. She unloads all over you. She pours out her heart and implores you to do something about "Suzie."

Then you go find Suzie and bring her to your office. You question her about what has been reported to you. Of course she denies it and has a completely different perspective of what has happened. You are careful not to tell her who reported this issue to you, because that person has begged you not to let Suzie know she told on her. So now you are stuck. What do you do? You have already spent more than an hour on this interpersonal conflict between two employees, and you are not even close to a resolution. That is because you cannot solve other people's conflicts. It is impossible. Yet you think it is your job.

You tell Suzie to make sure she does not ever do again what she was accused of doing and denies she did. And you think you have done your job. Now Suzie guesses at who reported to you and, depending on her personality, either approaches that person in an angry manner or goes and tells everyone else that person ratted on her. So, the conflict that began as a small misunderstanding is now growing into a war where others are taking sides. Finally, it culminates in a shouting match between the two employees that is witnessed by the elders. Now you have to spend more time comforting the elders, doing an abuse investigation, and counseling the two employees. The one who brought the complaint to you in the first place gets mad at you for speaking with Suzie and quits her job. How is this working for you?

Managing conflict does not mean that you try to fix things for everyone. It means you create a safe place for people to resolve their own conflicts. It means that you educate everyone in a conflict resolution model that is simple to use. Then you train all of your managers in conflict mediation. There needs to be someone in your community who is a trained conflict mediator at all times. Then you raise the expectation. It is now the expectation that all conflict will be resolved in a professional manner before it bleeds over onto the heads of the elders.

We need to shift our beliefs around conflict. In a human community, there will be conflict. Count on it. You cannot change that. We are human. We have these large elephants (our emotional side). We also have these judging brains that judge ourselves differently than we judge others. We have these filters on our belief windows that color everything that happens. We are terrible at communication. That is a combination that leads to conflict. Although you cannot stop conflict from occurring, you can begin to see conflict as a means for building a high-trust environment. If it is managed properly, conflict can be a means for understanding each other better.

Once we have taught our managers how to mediate conflict, we have created a safe environment where people can resolve their own conflicts. We give our managers a brightly colored, laminated card with the conflict mediation model steps on one side and the ground rules for resolving conflict on the other. I love it when I go into one of our communities and see a manager walking down the hall with one of those cards in her hand. What a difference changing this one routine can have on the climate of the community, on the well-being of elders and staff, and on managers' lives! Seeing conflict as something normal that simply needs managing changes the context of your community.

These are life skills that your employees can take outside of their work life and carry into their personal lives. Leadership can and does change people's lives.

PRINCIPLES FOR ETHICAL DECISION MAKING

Another keystone habit that will help you change the culture of your community is developing your community's principles for ethical decision making. These are guidelines that can help you and everyone in your organization understand how you make decisions based upon ethical principles, not emotions.

Most people in your organization have never before been in a position of decision-making authority. They do not know how to make decisions as a formal leader. Many of them believe that you get to make decisions as a formal leader because you "feel like it." They are not privy to all of the information you have when you make a decision. They do not know the parameters that you have for making decisions. They do not know that sometimes you lie awake all night when you have a hard decision to make. Most do not realize how you cry sometimes over those decisions. In fact, they most likely have these filters on their belief window:

- Managers do not care about anything but money.

- Managers have their favorites who can do what they want to do.

- Managers make decisions without all of the information.

Have you even thought about what drives your decision making? If not, it is time to begin. Because you not only need to know what values are driving your own decision making, but you also need to empower teams to make decisions. And if you are using emotions to drive your decisions, you need to stop.

When you use emotional decision making, you create an unstable, uncertain climate. People cannot depend on or trust your decision making. You create uncertainty that leads to anxiety. You want to know that even when you are not in your community, everyone there knows how decisions are made and can make them the same way you would.

At Vivage, we have adopted a set of principles for ethical decision making within our community (they are shown in the box "Principles for Ethical Decision Making"). I share these with you as a model for developing your own principles that drive decision making in your community. They should be a reflection of the mission and values of your unique organization.

GOSSIP AND SOCRATES

The final keystone habit is also about how we create an ethos that supports the well-being of everyone in our community. One of the most destructive habits I have found in a community is the practice of unchecked gossip. People thrive on storytelling. And in the absence of a positive story to tell, they will resort to making stories up. When that happens, it can weaken, impede, and sometimes destroy any efforts for changing the culture of care.

Person-centered leaders need to gain the skills of storytelling. Human beings resonate with stories. They learn from stories. Having powerful, meaningful stories about your vision of creating a different world for your care community is essential.

Gossip is a form of storytelling that is designed to tear down, not build up. I have never heard anyone gossip about anything good. Gossip is typically telling stories about other people. These stories are often untrue, and they are intended to be divisive. Gossip runs rampant in our care communities.

Leaders can replace that habit by teaching everyone that we are acting in the best interest of the elders by not participating in gossip. It takes all of us, working together, to meet the needs of our elders. Gossip destroys the trust we need to do our sacred work.

We can look to Socrates for help in stopping the gossip. Because Socrates did not leave any of his ideas in written form, we only know about him through secondhand sources. The following fable is a popular one that is often attributed to him. You can use it as a tool to help show people that they do not need to participate in the destructive habit of gossiping.

Strong minds discuss ideas, average minds discuss events, weak minds discuss people. (Socrates)

The Triple Filter Test

One fine day, an acquaintance of Socrates came to see him. After a brief conversation, he said, "Do you know what I just heard about Diogenes?"

"Hold on a minute," Socrates retorted. "Before telling me anything, I'd like you to pass a little test. It's called the Triple Filter Test."

"Triple filter?"

"That is correct," Socrates remarked. "Before you talk to me about Diogenes, it might be a good idea to take a moment and filter what you're going to say. That's why I call it the triple filter test. The first filter is Truth. Have you made absolutely sure that what you are about to tell me about Diogenes is true?"

"No," the man said, "Actually I just heard about it and . . ."

"All right", said Socrates. "So you don't really know if it's true or not. Now let's try the second filter, the filter of Goodness. Is what you are about to tell me about my friend something good?"

"No, on the contrary."

"So", Socrates continued, "you want to tell me something bad about him, but you're not certain it's true. You may still pass the test though because there's one filter left: The filter of Usefulness. Is what you want to tell me about my friend going to be useful to me?"

"No, not really."

"Well", concluded Socrates, "if what you want to tell me is neither true nor good nor even useful, why tell it to me at all?"

Now you have seven keystone habits that you can use to dramatically change the culture and climate of your care community. I list them here, along with how they each motivate the elephant:

1. *Daily community meetings:* Give the elders a voice

2. *Learning circles and huddles:* Give everyone an equal voice

3. *Cohesive leadership team:* Presents a unified voice from the leaders

4. *Code of conduct:* Sets the standards of conduct that elders determine for their home

5. *Managing conflict:* Creates a safe place for everyone

6. *Principles of ethical decision making:* Creates security that decisions are made by principle instead of emotions

7. *Managing gossip:* Creates an environment of trust

Who could argue that any of these new habits are not worth pursuing? Implementing these routines will start an evolution of change in your community that will be difficult to stop. The only ones who can stop an evolution are the leaders. You are also the ones who can start it and keep it going.

Principles for Ethical Decision Making

All team and individual decision making should be made on an ethical basis, not an emotional basis. The following principles guide us in our mission and our work where service, innovation, and profitability are woven together to create a caring community.

1. Is this what is best for the organization and our customers?
   - Will this decision negatively impact our mission or those we serve?
   - Are we ensuring the quality of service that sets us apart?
   - Are we meeting all of our contractual and ethical obligations?
   - Does this decision reflect the values and priorities of the organization?

Examples of decision making that meet this principle:

   a. In deciding on their vacation and time-off schedules, the team ensures that there is ample coverage to provide back-up for our customers.
   b. Creating personal boundaries that ensure we can continue to hold others accountable to maintain the highest expectations of those we mentor and serve.

2. Is this fair to everyone?
   - Are we considering everyone's needs in making this decision?
   - Is this decision free from bias, impartiality, or injustice?
   - Does everyone on the team feel a sense of equity?

Examples of decision making that meet this principle:

   a. Being careful not to create cliques that exclude members of the team or prevent new employees from being included in team process.
   b. Ensuring each team member is treated evenly in scheduling work, travel, holidays, and vacations.

3. Is this consistent?
   - Is this consistent with past decisions we have made?
   - If we are faced with this decision in the future, will we be able to make the same decision?

Example of decision making that would meet this principle:

   a. The team holds one member accountable for too many absences. Six months later, another team member is facing family problems and will need to be absent a large amount of time. The team must also hold this person accountable by asking her to take some family leave time.

(continued)

(continued)

4. Is this fiscally responsible?
    *   Have we considered the financial implications of this decision?
    *   Are we convinced that any negative financial ramifications from this decision are outweighed by the ethical objective or long-term well-being of the organization?
    *   Is there a better way to do this that would not fiscally impact the organization in a negative way?

Examples of decision making that meet this principle:

a. The team ensures that in setting their schedules for time off that it does not create a situation where the organization may be penalized financially for that decision (i.e., during audit time when the organization would have to pay more to the auditing firm or by incurring unnecessary overtime)

b. The team ensures that its reports are completed in a timely manner; giving the homes information that can help them be more fiscally proactive.

5. Is this legal?
    *   Have we ensured that the decision we are making is within the law?
    *   Does this decision infringe on anyone's legal rights?
    *   Does this decision put the organization at risk legally?

Examples of decision making that meet this principle:

a. A member of the team is taking time off under the Family and Medical Leave Act. The team needs this person, but does not ask her to return to work early and forgo her benefits.

b. The team ensures that each member's actions within a home are always consistent with state and federal regulations.

c. The team ensures that any documents or printed material it uses maintain copyright laws and have gone through the organization's approval process.

Epilogue

The rewards for shifting beliefs, changing the context, and replacing routines will be many. Understanding the science of leadership and using it to elevate the art of your own leadership is the pathway to a sustainable, caring community where people want to live and work.

I wish you the best on this journey. Never forget that your work is sacred. Through your leadership you will change many lives.

References

Ariely, D. (2013). What motivates us at work? More than money. Retrieved from http://blog.ted.com/2013/04/10/what-motivates-us-at-work-7-fascinating-studies-that-give-insights/

Arnsten, A. F. T. (2009). Stress signalling pathways that impair prefrontal cortex structure and function. In *Nature Reviews Neuroscience* 10, 410–422. doi:10.1038/nrn2648.

Barsade, S. (2002). The ripple effect: Emotional contagion and its influence on group behavior. *Administrative Sciences Quarterly*, 47(4), 644–675.

Bennington, V. (n.d). The ups and downs of cortisol: What you need to know. Retrieved from http://breakingmuscle.com/health-medicine/the-ups-and-downs-of-cortisol-what-you-need-to-know

Bradberry, T. (2016). 9 things that make good employees quit. Retrieved from http://www.talentsmart.com/articles/9-Things-That-Make-Good-Employees-Quit-172420765-p-1.html

Brooks, D. (2011). *The Social Animal*. New York: Random House.

Browning, R. (2016). Retrieved from quotesthoughtsrandom.wordpress.com

Bruhn, J., & Wolf, S. (1979). *The Roseto Story: An Anatomy of Health*. Norman: University of Oklahoma Press.

Bruner, J. (1996). *The Culture of Education*. Cambridge, MA: Harvard University Press.

Cacioppo, J., Gardner, W., & Bernston, G. (1997). Beyond bipolar conceptualization and measures: The case of attitudes and evaluative space. *Personality and Social Psychology Review*, 1(1), 3–25.

Casey, J. (2016). Retrieved from www.casey.org/our-founder/

Certified Eden Associate Training Educator's Guide. (2015). Rochester, NY: The Eden Alternative.

Clarke, B. (2016). Retrieved from govleaders.org/quotes.htm

Covey, S.M. (2006). *The Speed of Trust: The One Thing that Changes Everything*. New York: Free Press.

D'Angelo, A. (2016). Retrieved from https://www.brainyquote.com/search_results.html?q=Without+a+sense+of+caring%2C+there+can+be+no

De Unamuno, M. (1925). *Essays and Soliloquies*. New York: Alfred A Knopf.

Dobda, E. (2016). Retrieved from www.goodreads.com/quotes/tag/paradigm-shift

Duhigg, C. (2012). *The Power of Habit: Why We Do What We Do in Life and Business*. New York: Random House.

Drummond, N. (2016). Retrieved from www.quantisoft.com/Articles/Quotes.htm#sl

Dyer, W. (2015). Dr. Wayner Dyer lives on. Retrieved from http://www.huffingtonpost.com

Eaton, S. (2001). What a difference management makes! Nursing staff turnover variation within a single labor market. Appropriateness of Minimum Nurse Staffing Ratios in Nursing Homes CMS Phase II Final Report.

ERC. (2014). What is organizational climate? Retrieved from https://www.yourerc.com/blog/post/What-is-Organizational-Climate.aspx

Etheridge, M. 2006. I need to wake up. From the album *The Road Less Travelled*. BMG Rights Management.

Exline, J., & Hill, P. (2012). Humility: a consistent and robust predictor of generosity. *Journal of Positive Psychology*, (7), 208–218.

Farrell, D., Brady, C., & Frank, B. (2011). *Meeting the Leadership Challenge in Long-Term Care: What You Do Matters*. Baltimore, MD: Health Professions Press.

Forbes-Thompson, S., Leiker, T., & Bleich, M. R. (2007). High performing and low-performing nursing homes: A view from complexity science. *Health Care Management Review, 32*(4), 341–351.

Foster, D. (2016). Retrieved from http://davidfoster.tv/10-signs-you%E280%99 re-living-in-lala-land/

Fox, N. (2007). *The Journey of a Lifetime: Leadership Pathways to Culture Change in Long-Term Care*. Milwaukee, WI: Action Pact

Fox, N., Norton, L., Ransom, S., Tellis-Nayak, V., Brostsoki, D., Tellis-Nayak, M., Beatty, S., Grant, L., Dean, S., & Thomas, W. (2005). *Well-being: Beyond Quality of Life, the Metamorphosis of Eldercare*. Milwaukee, WI: Action Pact

Frank, B. (2016). Harnessing insights on interpersonal relationships and organizational cultures to improve staff stability. Presentation at AHCA-NCAL Quality Summit, San Antonio, TX.

Freeman, J., Stolier, R., Ingbretsen, Z., & Hehman, E. (2014). Amygdala responsivity to high-level social information from unseen forces. *The Journal of Neuroscience, 34*(32), 10573–10581.

Gilbert, S. (1997). A nursing home? Or death? Retrieved from http://www.nytimes.com/1997/08/06/us/a-nursing-home-or-death.html

Gladwell, M., (2006). *The Tipping Point: How Little Things Can Make a Big Difference*. New York: Hachette Book Group.

Haidt, J. (2006). *The Happiness Hypothesis: Finding Modern Truth in Ancient Wisdom*. New York: Basic Books.

Hanson, R. (2009). *Buddha's Brain*. Oakland, CA: New Harbinger Publications.

Heath, C., & Heath, D. (2010). *Switch: How to Change Things When Change Is Hard*. New York: Crown Business.

Higgins, B., & Bergman, C. (2011). *The Everything Guide to Evidence of the Afterlife: A Scientific Approach to Proving the Existence of Life After Death*. Fairfield, OH: Adams Media.

Irving, J. (2016). Retrieved from www.inspirationalquotestoday.com/2012/03/inspirational-quote-from-john-irving.html

Isen, A. (2001). An influence of positive affect on decision making in complex situations: Theoretical issues and implications. *Journal of Consumer Psychology, 11*(2), 75–85.

James Bird Guess International Success Academy. (2016). Worst performing leaders: 5 qualities that define them. Retrieved from http://internationalsuccessacademy.com/worst-performing-leaders-5-qualities-that-define-them

Kahneman, D. (2011). *Thinking Fast and Slow*. New York: Farrar, Straus and Giroux.

Kaku, M. (2016). Retrieved from https://globaldigitalcitizen.org/40-leaning-quotes

Kay, J. (1993). *How Business Strategies Add Value*. New York: Oxford University Press.

Kayser-Jones, J., Schell, E., & Kramer, A. M. (1997). The effect of staffing on the quality of care at mealtime. *Nursing Outlook, 45*(2), 64–71.

King, M. L. Jr., & King, C. S. (2002). *Martin Luther King: In My Own Words*. London: Hodder & Staughton.

Kouzes, J. (2000). Link me to your leader. *Business 2.0*.

Kramer, A. M., & Fish, R. (2001). The relationship between nurse staffing levels and the quality of nursing home care. Appropriateness of Minimum Nurse Staffing Ratios in Nursing Homes, Phase II Final Report. Washington, DC: U.S. Department of Health and Human Services, Health Care Financing Administration.

Kratzer, C. C. (1997). Case study: Roscoe Elementary School: Cultivating a caring community in an urban elementary school. *Journal of Education for Students Place at Risk, 2*(4), 345–375.

Leape, L. (2000). Patient safety. Medical errors: Hearings before the Committee on Health, Education, Labor and Pensions, Senate, 106th Congress, January 26.

Lencioni, P. (2005). *Overcoming the Five Dysfunctions of a Team: A Field Guide for Leaders, Managers and Facilitators*. San Francisco: Jossey-Bass.

Lescoe-Long, M., & Long, M. (1998). Identifying behavior change intervention points to improve staff retention in nursing homes. Report and recommendations to the Kansas Association of Homes and Services for the Aging.

Lindbergh, A. M. (2005). *Gift from the Sea*. New York: Random House.

Marx, D. (2007). Patient safety and a just culture. Retrieved from http://www.unmc.edu/patient-safety/_documents/patient-safety-and-the-just-culture.pdf

McGregor, D. (1960). *The Human Side of Enterprise*. New York: McGraw-Hill.

McWilliams, P. (2016). Retrieved from https://www.askideas.com/if-you-change-the-belief-first-changing-the-action-is-easier/

Mitchell, J. (1967). Both sides now. From the album *Clouds*. Reprise Records.

Mullainathan, W., & Shafir, E. (2013). *Scarcity: Why Having Too Little Means So Much*. New York: Times Books.

Norton, L. (2016). Learning circles. Retrieved from http://actionpact.com/resources/the_learning_circle

Pascotto, V., Goddard, J., & Gallwey, T. (2010). A workplace consonant with human values. *Interconnections, Issue 5*.

Payne, R. K., & DeVol, P. E. (2006). *Bridges Out of Poverty: Strategies for Professionals and Communities*. Highlands, TX: aha! Process, Inc.

Piff, P. K., Stancato, D. M., Côté, S., Mendoza-Denton, R., & Keltner, D. (2012). Higher social class predicts increased unethical behavior. *Proceedings of the National Academy of Sciences, 109*(11), 4086–4091. doi:10.1073/pnas.1118373109

Pink, D. (2009). *Drive: The Surprising Truth About What Motivates Us*. New York: Riverhead Books.

Popper, K. (1972). An approach to the problem of rationality and the freedom of man. *Objective Knowledge: An Evolutionary Approach*. New York: Oxford University Press.

Power, G. A. (2010). *Dementia Beyond Drugs: Changing the Culture of Care*. Baltimore, MD: Health Professions Press.

Power, G. A. (2014). *Dementia Beyond Disease: Enhancing Well-Being*. Baltimore, MD: Health Professions Press.

Putnam, R. D. (2000). *Bowling Alone*. New York: Simon & Schuster.

Rain, J. (2016). Retrieved from http://asquote.com/quote/tag/path?page=15

Risley, T. R., & Hart, B. (1995). *Meaningful Differences in the Everyday Experience of Young American Children*. Baltimore: Paul H. Brookes Publishing.

Ryan, P. (2016). Retrieved from http://www.brainyquote.com/quotes/p/paulryan440783.html?scr=t_community

Sandrone, V. (1997). F. W. Taylor and scientific management. Retrieved from http://www.skymark.com/resources/leaders/taylor.asp

Schneider, S., Ehrhart, M., & Macey, W. (2013). Organizational climate and culture. *Annual Review of Psychology* (64), 361–388. doi: 10.1146/annurev-psych-113011-143809

Scioli, A., & Biller, H. (2010). *The Power of Hope: Overcoming Your Most Daunting Life Difficulties—No Matter What*. Deerfield Beach, FL: Health Communications, Inc.

Shields, S., & Norton, L. (2006). *In Pursuit of the Sunbeam: A Practical Guide to Transformation from Institution to Household*. Milwaukee, WI: Action Pact.

Singer, T. (2012). The perfect amount of stress. *Psychology Today*. Retrieved from https://www.psychologytoday.com/articles/201203/the-perfect-amount-stress

Smith, H. (2013). *The Power of Perception: 6 Steps to Behavior Change*. Juxtabook Digital Marketing.

Socrates. Retrieved from https://www.quora.com/What-is-Triple-Filter-test-of-Socrates

Stroebel, R. (2014). The Eden Alternative in South Africa: Exploring personhood and identity within a unique cultural context. Concurrent session, 7th Eden Alternative International Conference, Nashville, TN.

Sunnubian. (2014). Shikoba Nabajyotisaikia! [Is This The Answer?]. Retrieved from http://www.africanamerica.org/topic/shikoba-nabajyotisaikia-is-this-the-answer

Suttle, E. (2013). Increasing your leadership influence in long term care. Closing plenary, Colorado Heath Care Association Fall Conference, Denver.

Tannen, D. (1991). Men and women use different approaches in classroom discussion. Retrieved from http://www.chronicle.com/article/MenWomen-Use-Different/87336.

Taylor, S. E. (1991). Asymmetrical effects of positive and negative events: The mobilization—minimization hypothesis. *Psychological Bulletin*, 110, 67–85.

Thomas, W. H. (1999). *The Eden Alternative handbook*. Sherburne, NY: Summer Hill Company, Inc.

Thomas, W. H. (2004). *What Are Old People For? How Elders Will Save the World*. Acton, MA: Vanderwyk & Burnham.

Todorov, A., Baron, S. G., & Oosterhof, N. N. (2008). Evaluating face trustworthiness: A model based approach. *Social Cognitive and Affective Neuroscience, 3*(2), 119–127. http://doi.org/10.1093/scan/nsn009

Tomasello, M., Melis, A., Tennie, C., Wyman, E., & Herrmann, E. (2012). Two key steps in the evolution of human cooperation: The interdependence hypothesis. *Current Anthropology, 53*(6), 673.

Transparency Market Research. (2015). Global anti-aging market boosted by baby boomer population nearing retirement. Retrieved from http://www.transparencymarketresearch.com/pressrelease/anti-aging-market.htm

Tutu Foundation. (2016). Retrieved from http://www.tutufoundationuk.org/about

Twain, M. (1905). *The Refuge of the Derelicts*. Unpublished manuscript.

Vohs, K., Glass, B., Maddox, W., & Markman, A. (2011). Ego depletion is not just fatigue: Evidence from a total sleep deprivation experiment. *Social Psychology and Personality Science, 2*(2), 166–173.

Wheatley, M. (2010). Some friends and I started talking. Retrieved from http://www.mindful.org/some-friends-and-i-started-talking/

Williams, R. (1995). Self-directed work teams: A competitive advantage. Retrieved from http://www.qualitydigest.com/magazine/1995/nov/article/self-directed-work-teams-competitive-advantage.html#

Wise, R. A. (2011). *Wise Quotes of Wisdom: A Lifetime Collection of Quotes, Sayings, Philosophies, Viewpoints and Thoughts.* Bloomington, IN: AuthorHouse Publishing.

Index

Note: *b* indicates boxes, *f* indicates figures, *t* indicates tables.